Medical Coding for Non-Coders

Second Edition

Karen S. Scott,
MEd, RHIA, CCS-P, CPC

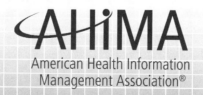

American Health Information
Management Association®

ISBN: 978-1-58426-081-3
AHIMA Product No.: AC202213

AHIMA Staff:
Ann Barta, MSA, RHIA, CDIP, Director, HIM Practice Excellence
Jessica Block, MA, Assistant Editor
Megan Grennan, Production Development Editor
Jason Malley, Creative Content Director
Pamela Woolf, Managing Editor

For more information about AHIMA Press publications, including updates, visit http://www.ahima.org/publications/updates.aspx

American Health Information Management Association
233 North Michigan Avenue, 21st Floor
Chicago, Illinois 60601-5809
ahima.org

Contents

About the Author   v

Preface   vii

Acknowledgments   ix

Foreword   xi

Chapter One: Overview of Coding Systems   1

Coding Defined and Explained	1
International Classification of Diseases, Tenth Revision, Clinical Modification	4
International Classification of Diseases, Tenth Revision, Procedure Classification System	13
Overview of ICD-9-CM	17
Other Issues in Coding Diagnoses	17
Medical Necessity	18
Revisions to ICD-10	19
ICD-11	19
Healthcare Common Procedure Coding System	20
Current Procedural Terminology	23

Chapter Two: Reimbursement Overview   33

Medicare	33
Other Medicare Inpatient PPSs	43
Ambulatory Payment Classifications (APCs): Medicare Outpatient PPS	45
Payment for Physicians: Resource-Based Relative Value System/Scale	52
Other Insurance Programs	54

Commercial and Nonprofit Group Medical
  Insurance Plans   56
Forms Overview: Billing Forms and Their
  Components and Fields Explained   57

Chapter Three: Coding Compliance 61

Fraud and Abuse   61
Recovery Audit Contractors (RACs)   64
Standards of Ethical Coding   64
Policies and Procedures   64
Components of a Compliance Plan   65
Healthcare Quality Improvement Organizations   69

Chapter Four: Other Issues Impacting Coding 73

The Coding Process   73
Quality Assessment for the Coding Process   79
Coding Professionals   83
Coding Technology   86

References   89
APPENDIX A   91
APPENDIX B   101
Index   113

About the Author

Karen S. Scott, MEd, RHIA, CCS-P, CPC, has more than 20 years of experience in the healthcare field. Ms. Scott is the sole proprietor of Karen Scott Seminars and Consulting. She has been an educator for many years including teaching in the Health Information Management Programs at the University of Tennessee Health Science Center and Arkansas Tech University. She has worked as an HIM director in an acute care hospital setting, training director for a national transcription company, and reimbursement specialist for a regional physicians' group. She holds a bachelor of science degree in Health Information Management and a master's degree of education in Instructional Technology from Arkansas Tech University in Russellville, Arkansas. She is past-president of both the Tennessee and Arkansas Health Information Management Associations and is a past-chair of the AHIMA Council on Certification. She serves as a commissioner on the Commission on Accreditation of Health Informatics and Information Management (CAHIIM). Ms. Scott has won several awards, including the Tennessee Innovator Award and the Distinguished Member Award.

Ms. Scott teaches seminars on coding, reimbursement, medical terminology, and management throughout the country for physician and hospital audiences. She has published numerous articles on various healthcare topics including chapters in HIM and coding textbooks. Ms. Scott is author of the AHIMA textbook, *Coding and Reimbursement for Hospital Inpatient Services.*

Preface

Today's healthcare environment is complex, and the coding process is a fundamental part of the healthcare delivery system. It is imperative that those seeking to become versed in healthcare delivery also understand coding procedures and the impact that coding has on this delivery system.

Medical Coding for Non-Coders offers the reader an explanation and appreciation for the role that coding plays in the overall reimbursement system. It provides a basis for timely topics such as compliance and ethical issues that are common in today's healthcare system.

This text is a valuable resource for all members of the healthcare administrative team who regularly communicate with coding department managers and coders. Others associated with healthcare delivery would also benefit from understanding how the documentation they supply impacts the coding process and, therefore, healthcare data, and reimbursement as a whole.

Chapter 1 provides an overview of the coding system. Chapter 2 discusses reimbursement. Chapter 3 explains coding compliance, and chapter 4 addresses other issues that impact coding. The two appendices following the text provide the AHIMA standards of ethical coding and steps for managing an effective query process.

Melinda A. Wilkins, PhD., RHIA
Program Director and Professor
Arkansas Tech University

Acknowledgments

The author would like to thank Susan Parker, MEd, RHIA, and Melinda A. Wilkins, PhD., MEd, RHIA, for their contributions to this publication. The author expresses appreciation to Claudia A. Potts, MSM, RHIT, for her review of this edition.

Foreword

This book is a must read by healthcare professionals in all contexts. It provides an unparalleled resource for anyone in today's healthcare industry. Ms. Scott carefully and thoroughly walks the reader through the maze of terms and provides a clear explanation that will give the reader confidence in their ability to understand coding, its significance, and the terminology surrounding it. Although several resources exist, this is the one book destined to be on the shelf in every department involved in healthcare.

Changing reimbursement systems, meaningful use, HIPAA regulations, and a completely new coding system have created a challenging environment for healthcare providers. Ms. Scott's new book takes the mystery out of it. She explains the new *International Classification of Diseases, Tenth Revision* by providing crosswalks and examples. She guides the reader through the reimbursement system at the appropriate level of proficiency, without weighing one down with unnecessary information or attempting to create a textbook for coders.

The book should be the go to resource for new graduates as well as seasoned administrators who require a clearer understanding of issues impacting the bottom line. The chapters cover all the bases, from payers needs to computer-assisted coding, and the effects of new regulations.

From the very outset, she explains the basics of coding and helps the reader develop an understanding without tackling the intricacies that often drive non-coders away. The book simplifies the acronyms and multiple coding systems by clearly explaining the function and distinction between each.

Ms. Scott builds on a foundation of distinguishing between coding and reimbursement. The book is an excellent resource for those who need to understand coding for payment and those who use coded data for statistics and research.

Anyone in outcomes management, quality, compliance, revenue cycle, or consulting will find the overview of compliance a well-written and illustrative guide for facility success. It contains explanations on monitoring, internal quality indicators, how to spot important patterns, and why they matter.

This resource provides an ethical template for all coders as well as the finer points of how to query physicians regarding documentation and clarification. Big data are driven, in part, by the codes and the clinical documentation supporting them. Ms. Scott's book transcends specific job titles and focuses on the uniform need for all healthcare workers to have a clear foundational understanding of coding and the related areas. This book does that exceptionally well.

Susan Parker, MEd, RHIA
President, Seagate Consultants

Susan Parker is a seasoned Health Information Management professional. She has served in many national offices including being elected as the American Health Information Management Association's very first Speaker of the House in 2012. Ms. Parker is a published author and speaker on the subject of Health Information Management and Innovation. For the past 22 years, Ms. Parker has been the President of Seagate Consultants, a Recruitment Firm focusing on Health Information Management careers. Susan Parker can be reached at seagatejobs@bellsouth.net or www.seagateconsultants.com.

Overview of Coding Systems

Coding of medical records has been a stable function in the health information management field for many years. In the mid-1980s when the federal government decided to base inpatient Medicare reimbursement on coded data, this function took on greater importance. Since that time, nearly all Medicare reimbursement in all settings is tied to coded diagnoses and procedures. Most insurance companies base their reimbursement on these codes as well, so understanding how medical codes are assigned and how they are used in the various reimbursement processes is vital to the understanding of reimbursement. This book explains the basics of coding and helps readers become more proficient in their understanding of coding without actually turning them into coding professionals (coders).

Coding Defined and Explained

Although coding is used in many different ways, for the purpose of this book, medical "coding" is the assignment of a universal number to diagnoses and procedure descriptions. The code numbers are very detailed to be able to describe the diagnoses (what is wrong with the patient) and the procedures performed to test or correct these diagnoses. Because medicine is not always an exact science, codes have been developed to identify all reasons for seeking healthcare, including an annual physical examination or the need to become vaccinated against diseases.

It is important to understand that coding is not just used for reimbursement. The most important use of coded data is for patient care.

Physicians and other healthcare practitioners can use codes to identify symptoms that need to be evaluated and alert other healthcare professionals to life-threatening conditions. Codes are also used to help with administrative functions such as staffing, scheduling, and adding or decreasing healthcare services. In many states, codes are used along with other healthcare statistics to compare facilities and plan for new services for underserved areas.

Over the years, diseases and medical-surgical procedures have come to be known by different names. For example, Down syndrome is sometimes referred to as mongolism or trisomy 21. Clearly, the use of more than one term for the same disease makes it difficult to collect and retrieve information. In an effort to organize and standardize medical language, the healthcare industry has developed nomenclatures, classification systems, and clinical vocabularies. These systems facilitate the organization, storage, and retrieval of healthcare diagnostic and procedural data. Moreover, they aid in the development and implementation of computerized patient record systems.

Coding Data Sets

The Health Insurance Portability and Accountability Act (HIPAA) of 1996 required the establishment of electronic transactions and coding standards. In 2000, the Department of Health and Human Services (HHS), in accordance with HIPAA, established official medical coding set standards. To be in compliance with the HIPAA law, all covered entities are required to use the following official medical coding sets:

- *International Classification of Diseases, Tenth Revision, Clinical Modification (ICD-10-CM)* is the system that is used for reporting all diseases, injuries, impairments, other health problems and causes of such, and *International Classification of Diseases, Tenth Revision, Procedure Coding System (ICD-10-PCS)* is used to report procedures performed on hospital inpatients and claims for discharges or dates of service after October 1, 2014. Before this date, they were coded with the ICD-9-CM system that was the official coding set before the transition to ICD-10.

- Healthcare Common Procedure Coding System (HCPCS), which includes Current Procedural Terminology (CPT) is used for reporting physician and other healthcare services, including all outpatient procedures.

- Current Dental Terminology (CDT), Code on Dental Procedures and Nomenclatures is used for reporting dental services.

- National Drug Codes (NDC) were designated, in the original ruling from Medicare, as the official data set for reporting drugs used by pharmacies. However, this adoption was repealed in 2003. Currently, there is no official standard for reporting medications on pharmacy transactions.

HIPAA does not allow for overlapping data sets. This requires all users of the coding system to adopt the most updated version on the same date. For example, ICD-10-CM changes become effective each year on October 1. This aspect of the law requires all users to adopt the changes effective with discharges or services rendered on or after the October 1 deadline.

As of October 1, 2014, the main coding systems used in the United States for healthcare reporting are ICD-10-CM, ICD-10-PCS, HCPCS, and CPT. ICD-10-CM is used in all healthcare settings for diagnosis coding. The ICD-10-PCS consists of procedures used for hospital inpatient billing only. The other main system used, HCPCS, is made up of two levels of codes. The base level, or level I HCPCS codes, is *CPT*, published each year by the American Medical Association (AMA). The second level, or national code set, is HCPCS Level II codes, which are mainly used for Medicare reimbursement; however, most insurance plans do accept some HCPCS Level II Codes.

Before October 1, 2014, HIPAA required that ICD-9-CM diagnosis and procedure codes be used for hospital inpatients and that ICD-9-CM diagnosis codes and CPT/HCPCS procedure codes be used for ambulatory patients, laboratory and radiology services, and physicians' professional billing. Beginning with discharges and dates of service on October 1, 2014, ICD-10-CM will be the official data set for coding diagnoses in all healthcare settings. ICD-10-PCS will be utilized to code and report inpatient procedures by hospitals. This transition will not impact coding procedures with CPT/HCPCS coding sets as ICD-10 will not replace CPT/HCPCS. It is possible that prior claims will be reviewed by Medicare contractors and other agencies for several years after this transition. Since audits may reach back to previous cases of up to five years, knowledge of the legacy system of ICD-9-CM will be essential to resolve billing issues and address allegations of improper coding and billing. Facilities should maintain access to ICD-9 information and guidance to assist reviews of older claims.

International Classification of Diseases, Tenth Revision

One coding system of importance is the *International Statistical Classification of Diseases and Related Health Problems, Tenth Revision (ICD-10)*. Established by the World Health Organization (WHO), the ICD system was designed to be totally revised at 10-year intervals. In the mid-1990s, WHO published the newest version of ICD, *International Statistical Classification of Diseases and Related Health Problems, Tenth Revision*, known as ICD-10. This revision is currently in use by many countries throughout the world and has been used in the United States to capture mortality statistics since 1999. However, studies in the United States determined that ICD-10 needed to be modified to capture data that would support the reimbursement system before the implementation; hence, it was modified to become ICD-10-CM. ICD-10-CM does not include a procedure section; hence, ICD-10-PCS was developed to capture procedures performed in the inpatient hospital setting.

International Classification of Diseases, Tenth Revision, Clinical Modification (ICD-10-CM)

The ICD-10-CM code book is updated every year with changes effective October 1 of that year. These updates are known as the Addenda. It is essential that code books and coding software be updated yearly with the revisions. Many code books come in a loose leaf version with updates provided at an extra charge. Encoders and other electronic coding software are typically updated on a quarterly basis to include all current changes. ICD-10-CM was not developed for use as a reimbursement system, even though it is now the basis for hospital reimbursement within the diagnosis-related group (DRG) system (see Chapter 2). It was designed for statistical collection. It is a classification system, which means codes are grouped together into various classes based on clinical information and body systems.

Purpose

Coding is utilized for many purposes, some of these are as follows:

- Classifying morbidity and mortality information for statistical purposes
- Indexing hospital records by disease and operations
- Reporting diagnoses by physicians
- Storing and retrieving data
- Reporting national morbidity and mortality data
- Serving as the basis of DRG assignment for hospital reimbursement
- Reporting and compiling healthcare data to assist in the evaluation of medical care planning for healthcare delivery systems
- Determining patterns of care among healthcare providers
- Analyzing payments for health services
- Conducting epidemiological and clinical research

The Cooperating Parties

ICD-10-CM is maintained by four organizations known as the Cooperating Parties:

- National Center for Health Statistics (NCHS)
- American Hospital Association (AHA)
- American Health Information Management Association (AHIMA)
- Centers for Medicare and Medicaid Services (CMS)

Primarily, NCHS is responsible for updating the ICD-10-CM diagnosis classification and CMS is responsible for updating ICD-10-PCS.

AHIMA works to help provide training and certification, and AHA maintains the Central Office on ICD-10-CM and publishes *Coding Clinic for ICD-10-CM* and *ICD-10-PCS*, which contains the official coding guidelines and official guidance on the usage of ICD-10-CM and ICD-10-PCS. In 1985, the Coordination and Maintenance Committee was established. Co-chaired by representatives of NCHS and CMS, the committee is made up of advisors and representatives of all the Cooperating Parties. It meets twice a year to provide a public forum for discussing possible revisions and updates to ICD-10. Discussions at these meetings are advisory only. The director of NCHS and the administrator of CMS determine all final revisions. Coding advice is approved by CMS for Medicare reimbursement and accepted by many other healthcare plans, Medicaid programs, and state data sets. *Coding Clinic* is published quarterly and includes discussion of selected questions from the coding community along with guidance on how to appropriately assign codes for the scenarios discussed in the specific questions and should be utilized for coding by hospitals, outpatient and ambulatory services, physician professional services and other healthcare settings.

AHA's Central Office serves as the official US clearing house on medical coding for the proper use of the ICD-9-CM systems and Level I HCPCS (CPT-4 codes) for hospital providers and certain Level II HCPCS codes for hospitals, physicians, and other healthcare professionals. This office also serves in a representation and advocacy role on national classification and data issues.

Official ICD-10-CM Coding Guidelines

It is important to note that a hierarchy exists regarding rules and regulations for correct usage of ICD-10-CM. First, the coding professional must check all guidelines, rules, and notes found in the code book. For further instructions on code usage, the coder should review the official coding guidelines and *Coding Clinic* to ensure all official guidance has been followed.

Included in the HIPAA regulations for medical code data sets was the requirement that all users of ICD-10-CM must follow the official coding guidelines. These guidelines contain both general and chapter-specific guidelines as well as guidelines for inpatient and outpatient settings, such as physician practice and outpatient hospital settings. The official coding guidelines are divided into four main sections:

Section I: Conventions, general coding guidelines, and chapter-specific guidelines (this section is applicable to all healthcare settings unless otherwise indicated).

Section II: Selection of principal diagnosis (this section is applicable to all inpatient settings including acute, short term, long-term care, psychiatric hospitals, home health agencies, rehabilitation facilities, and nursing homes).

Section III: Reporting additional diagnoses (this section is applicable to all inpatient settings including acute, short-term, and long-term care, psychiatric hospitals, home health agencies, rehabilitation facilities, and nursing homes).

Section IV: Diagnostic coding and reporting guidelines for outpatient services (this section is applicable to hospital-based outpatient services and provider-based office visits).

It is important that all users of ICD-10-CM be aware of these rules and guidelines. It is recommended that they be implemented as part of the facility compliance program to ensure that all parties involved with coding and billing are referencing these rules as needed. Before being required by HIPAA law, these guidelines were not uniformly followed by some insurance companies and facilities. There have been instances where insurance companies have denied claims based on their internal coding guidelines that did not adhere to official coding guidelines. Facility contracts have included language that was contradictory to the coding guidelines. Denials and contract discrepancies should be reviewed carefully to check for these types of errors. Official coding guidelines for ICD-10-PCS were developed and should be utilized to assist in the training and transition process to the new coding systems.

Transition from ICD-9-CM to ICD-10-CM

The HHS published a final rule adopting ICD-10-CM (and ICD-10-PCS) to replace ICD-9-CM with the effective implementation date of October 1, 2013. This was delayed by final rule from October 1, 2013, to October 1, 2014.

Overview of Structure

Although the traditional ICD structure remains, ICD-10-CM is a complete alphanumeric coding scheme. The former supplementary classification information (V and E codes) was incorporated into the main classification system with different letters preceding the numerical portions of the codes. ICD-10 contains new chapters, and several categories have been restructured and new features added to maintain consistency with modern medicine. The disease classification has been expanded to provide greater specificity at the sixth digit level and with a seventh digit extension.

Examples of ICD-10-CM codes include the following:

- Malignant Neoplasm
  - C34.1   Malignant neoplasm of upper lobe, bronchus or lung
    - C34.10   Malignant neoplasm of upper lobe, unspecified bronchus or lung
    - C34.11   Malignant neoplasm of upper lobe, right bronchus or lung
    - C34.12   Malignant neoplasm of upper lobe, left bronchus or lung
- Diabetes
  - E10.2   Type 1 diabetes mellitus with kidney complications
    - E10.21   Type 1 diabetes mellitus with diabetic nephropathy

      Type 1 diabetes mellitus with intercapillary glomerulosclerosis

      Type 1 diabetes mellitus with intracapillary glomerulonephrosis

      Type 1 diabetes mellitus with Kimmelstiel-Wilson disease
    - E10.22   Type 1 diabetes mellitus with diabetic chronic kidney disease
    - E10.29   Type 1 diabetes mellitus with other diabetic renal complication

      Type 1 diabetes mellitus with renal tubular degeneration

How to Look Up a Term

Locating the correct and most specific code to identify the patient's medical condition is not as easy as just picking out a term in the code book. Several important steps are involved in the process. Each step must be carefully followed to allow for accurate coding.

Locating the Main Term

The first step is to look in the ICD-10-CM Alphabetic Index (Volume 2) under the main term. The main term is printed in bold type at the left margin, and is the main disease, injury, or condition causing the patient's symptoms. Examples of main terms are fracture, pneumonia, disease, injury, and enlarged. Anatomic terms (for example, kidney or shoulder) are *never* main terms in ICD-10-CM. If a coding professional tries to look up a code by the anatomic site, an instructional note to "see condition" will be found.

The Alphabetic Index is carefully cross-referenced to allow the coder to locate the correct code using several different terms. For example, the diagnosis "Barre-Guillain Syndrome" can be found under the main term "syndrome" as well as "Barre-Guillain." By looking up this diagnosis using either term, the coding professional is led to the correct code of G61.0.

Identify Subterms

Below the main terms are indented subterms that further describe the condition. They may describe different sites of the illness, etiology, or type of illness.

> **Bronchiolitis (acute) (infectious) (subacute) J21.9**
> with
> bronchospasm or obstruction J21.9
> influenza, flu, or grippe see influenza, with respiratory manifestations, NEC
> chemical J68.4

Nonessential Modifiers

Nonessential modifiers are terms in parentheses following main terms. These are modifiers or terms describing the main term whose presence or absence in the diagnostic statement does not change the code assignment. For example:

> **Intussusception (bowel) (colon) (enteric) (intestine) (rectum) K56.1**
> Appendix K38.8

Using the Tabular List (Volume 1)

Volume 2, the Alphabetic Index, leads the coder to the most likely code, but coding is not complete until the code is verified in the Tabular List found in Volume 1, called the ICD-10-CM Tabular List of Diseases and Injuries. In the Tabular List, codes are arranged numerically in 21 chapters and are grouped according to their cause (etiology), such as fractures, or body system (for example, digestive system).

Chapter titles in the ICD-10-CM are as follows:

1. Certain infectious and parasitic diseases
2. Neoplasms

3. Diseases of the blood and blood forming organs and certain disorders involving the immune mechanism
4. Endocrine, nutritional, and metabolic diseases
5. Mental, behavioral, and neurodevelopmental disorders
6. Diseases of the nervous system
7. Diseases of the eye and adnexa
8. Diseases of the ear and mastoid process
9. Diseases of the circulatory system
10. Diseases of the respiratory system
11. Diseases of the digestive system
12. Diseases of the skin and subcutaneous tissue
13. Diseases of the musculoskeletal system and connective tissue
14. Diseases of the genitourinary system
15. Pregnancy, childbirth and the puerperium
16. Certain conditions originating in the perinatal period
17. Congenital malformations, deformations, and chromosomal abnormalities
18. Symptoms, signs, and abnormal clinical and laboratory findings not elsewhere classified
19. Injuries, poisoning, and certain other consequences of external causes
20. External causes of morbidity
21. Factors influencing health status and contact with health services

The chapters are organized by type of condition and anatomical system. For example, Chapter 5, Mental, behavioral and neurodevelopmental disorders, represents a chapter that groups diseases by type of condition. Chapter 14, Diseases of the genitourinary system, represents a chapter that groups diseases by anatomical system.

Categories, Subcategories, and Subclassifications

ICD-10-CM is set up in categories and subcategories. Characters for these can be a combination of numbers or letters, but categories always begin with a letter. Categories are groups of three character codes made up of similar diseases or a single disease. Four or five character subcategories provide more information such as site of the illness, cause, or other characteristics of the disease. Codes can be from three to six characters long to provide even greater specificity. The coding professional must always code to the greatest level of specificity. Some codes will require a seventh character that identifies additional information such as the episode of care for an injury. If a code has less than six characters and requires a seventh character, a placeholder X is used to fill the spaces to make a valid seven character code. One example of this is V26.0 (motorcycle driver injured in a collision with other nonmotor vehicle in a nontraffic accident), which requires a seventh character to show the episode of care. To identify that this was the initial encounter, the correct code would be V26.0XXA.

Nonspecific or Residual Codes

ICD-10-CM allows for coding of all possible diagnoses and procedures. When the coder has a limited amount of information, a residual subcategory may be used. These include "other" and "unspecified" categories. The use of a residual subcategory should serve as a flag for the coding professional that a more specific code may be available to allow greater accuracy in code assignment. Although these residual codes are used appropriately in many instances, it should be noted that insurance companies are reviewing payment for codes that they consider "nonspecific." The coder should check the medical record and the code book for further clarification prior to assigning a nonspecific code. Many insurance companies also specify that some procedure codes are payable only with limited diagnoses. Many of the nonspecific codes are not on the "payable" diagnosis lists.

Coding Conventions

ICD-10-CM uses several terms, abbreviations, punctuations, and symbols to lead the coding professional to the correct codes. These coding conventions should be studied carefully and must be followed whenever present in the code book.

Square brackets [ ] are used in the tabular list to enclose synonyms, alternative wordings, and explanatory phrases, such as:

J00 Acute Nasopharyngitis [common cold]

The common cold is just another name for acute nasopharyngitis.

Square brackets can also be used to show that the number in the bracket can only be a manifestation and the other number must be assigned first as the underlying code or condition.

Nephropathy
    Sickle cell D57. – [N08]

Colons are used to show that there is an incomplete term that requires one or more of the terms after the colon to be present for the code to be used appropriately, for example:

N92.6 Irregular menstruation, unspecified

Excludes 1: *irregular menstruation with:*

lengthened intervals of scanty bleeding N91.3 – N91.5

shortened intervals of excessive bleeding N92.1

"See" and "see also" are terms that direct the coding professional to look under another main term if there is not enough information under the first term to identify the proper code.

Includes notes provide further examples or define the category:

S82 Fracture of lower leg, including ankle

Includes: *Fracture of malleolus*

There are two different types of Excludes notes in ICD-10-CM. Excludes 1 is a true exclude note. It means the diagnosis or symptom listed cannot be used in conjunction with the code:

G47.3 Sleep apnea

Code also any associated underlying condition
Excludes 1: *apnea NOS (R06.81)*
Cheyne-Stokes breathing (R06.3)
Pickwickian syndrome (E66.2)
Sleep apnea of newborn (P28.3)

Excludes 2 means that the diagnoses listed are not included in the code description so the coder may need to use two codes to fully capture the specificity in the diagnostic statement:

G47.6 Sleep related movement disorders

Excludes 2: *restless legs syndrome (G25.81)*

Notes appear in both the Tabular Lists and Alphabetic Indices to provide further instructions or give definitions. Notes are often used to help the coder translate physician terminology into coding terms.

"Code also" means the coding professional must use a second code to fully describe the condition. Sometimes the code book will instruct the coder to "use additional code to identify organism." This is instructing the coding professional to use an additional code to identify the organism if clear documentation in the chart shows a linkage between the diagnosis, such as urinary tract infection, stated to be caused by organisms such as *Escherichia coli* or *Streptococcus*:

N39.0 Urinary tract infection, site not specified

Use additional code (B95–B97), to identify infectious agent.

The code book does not always give hints, such as "use additional code" or "code also" to alert that more than one code is necessary. It is important that the coder use additional codes until all component parts of the diagnosis are fully described.

Not Elsewhere Classified and Not Otherwise Specified

NEC is an abbreviation that means not elsewhere classified. This means that a more specific category is not available in ICD-10-CM.

> **Pneumonia**
>> Bronchial
>>> Bacterial J15.9
>>>> Specified NEC J15.8

NOS stands for not otherwise specified. It should be interpreted as "unspecified" and is used when the coding professional has no further information available in the medical record to fully define the condition. H60.90 is unspecified otitis media, unspecified ear. Use this code when the diagnosis is identified as "otitis media" but is not specified as to type, severity, laterality, or manifestation.

Combination Codes

Many combination codes are provided in ICD-10-CM. For example, alcoholic cirrhosis is commonly found with the accompanying symptom of ascites. The code book allows for both the diagnosis and symptom to be coded with a single code:

K70.30 Alcoholic cirrhosis of liver without ascites

K70.31 Alcoholic cirrhosis of liver with ascites

Some coding professionals like to use a cheat sheet that lists many of the common diagnoses and procedures used in their facility or physician practices. Although a cheat sheet may save time in coding some diagnoses, it can also lead to many coding errors. Because ICD-10-CM does provide many combination codes that are to be used when two diagnoses are both present, if a coder is simply reading the code from a cheat sheet, the instructions to use combination codes will not be located. This is also true in the case of a physician simply checking off diagnoses from a fee ticket, superbill, or other standardized coding form.

Overall Steps of Coding

Every time a coding professional selects the appropriate code to describe the patient's diagnoses and procedures performed, he or she must go through the following steps:

1. Identify the main term(s) of the condition(s) to be coded.

2. Locate the main terms in the alphabetic index.

3. Refer to any subterms indented under the main term. This list may be extensive, so it is important that coders search the listing carefully. Also refer to any nonessential modifiers, instructional terms, or notes to select the most likely code.

4. Verify the code(s) in the tabular list.
5. Check all instructional terms in the tabular list and be sure to assign all codes to their highest degree of specificity.
6. Continue coding the diagnostic statement until all of the elements are identified completely.

It is important to understand that correct and accurate coding is a slow, thorough process. Documentation in the patient's health record must be reviewed carefully to ensure compliance with all rules, regulations, and guidelines impacting the code assignment. If ambiguous or unclear documentation is found, the coding professional must have a procedure in place to query the physician to clarify these points prior to code assignment.

Sequencing of Codes

Sequencing refers to the selection of the appropriate first diagnosis for the patient's encounter. For sequencing in the hospital inpatient and other inpatient settings, this first diagnosis is known as the principal diagnosis, which is the condition established after study to be chiefly responsible for occasioning the admission of the patient to the hospital for care as defined by the Uniform Hospital Discharge Data Set (UHDDS) guidelines. For example, if the patient was admitted for chest pain and after study it was found that the chest pain was caused by an acute myocardial infarction, the infarction would be the principal diagnosis. In the outpatient or physician office setting, the first listed diagnosis is sometimes known as the primary diagnosis and should be used in lieu of the principal diagnosis used in the outpatient setting. The first listed or primary diagnosis is the main reason—a symptom, chronic illness, or acute disease such as gastroenteritis or laceration—that caused the patient to seek treatment for that visit.

International Classification of Diseases, Tenth Revision, Procedure Classification System

ICD-10 does not include a procedure volume. Thus, when the United States began planning to clinically modify WHO's ICD-10, it was determined that creating a separate volume for procedures would be insufficient. As a result, CMS contracted with 3M Health Information Systems to develop a separate procedure code system that would serve as a replacement for ICD-9-CM, Volume 3. This coding system is known as the *International Classification of Diseases, 10th Revision, Procedure Classification System (ICD-10-PCS).*

Purpose and Use

According to CMS, the agency responsible for updating the procedure section of ICD-9-CM, the design of ICD-10-PCS included the following goals:

- Improve accuracy and efficiency of coding
- Reduce training effort
- Improve communication with physicians

ICD-10-PCS Coding Guidelines

Similar to the official coding guidelines for ICD-10-CM, the cooperating parties for the ICD-10-PCS, AHA, AHIMA, CMS, and NCHS have developed guidelines for usage of ICD-10-PCS that are based on the coding and sequencing instructions in ICD-10-PCS and are written to provide additional instruction. According to CMS,

> Adherence to these guidelines when assigning ICD-10-PCS procedure codes is required under the Health Insurance Portability and Accountability Act (HIPAA). The procedure codes have been adopted under HIPAA for hospital inpatient healthcare settings. A joint effort between the healthcare provider and the coder is essential to achieve complete and accurate documentation, code assignment, and reporting of diagnoses and procedures. These guidelines have been developed to assist both the healthcare provider and the coder in identifying those procedures that are to be reported. The importance of consistent, complete documentation in the medical record cannot be overemphasized. Without such documentation accurate coding cannot be achieved.

The guidelines are divided into sections including:

- Conventions
- Medical and Surgical Section Guidelines
  - o Body System
  - o Root Operation
  - o Body Part
  - o Approach
  - o Device
- Obstetrics Section Guidelines
- Other sections and guidelines will continue to be developed as needed.

Overview of Structure

ICD-10-PCS has no correlation to the ICD-10-CM structure. It consists of a multiaxial seven character alphanumeric code structure. Digits 0–9 and the alphabetic letters (A–H, J–N, and P–Z) are characters used in ICD-10-PCS. Although this system has the capability and flexibility to replace all existing procedural coding systems, it is currently being recommended to replace only ICD-9-CM procedure codes. Because of its unique structure, ICD-10-PCS is considered to be complete and expandable.

Because many different and confusing names of procedures are in use in the medical field, each root operation has been defined in ICD-10-PCS. This helps to clarify terms that currently have overlapping meaning, such as excision, resection, or removal.

Procedures are divided into 16 sections related to general type of procedure (medical and surgical, imaging, and so on):

Sections of ICD-10-PCS
0—Medical and Surgical
1—Obstetrics
2—Placement
3—Administration
4—Measurement and Monitoring
5—Extracorporeal Assistance and Performance
6—Extracorporeal Therapies
7—Osteopathic
8—Other Procedures
9—Chiropractic
B—Imaging
C—Nuclear Medicine
D—Radiation Therapy
F—Physical Rehabilitation and Diagnostic Audiology
G—Mental Health
H—Substance Abuse Treatment

All procedure codes have seven characters. The first character of the procedure code always specifies the section where the procedure is indexed. The second through seventh characters have a standard meaning within each section. In the Medical and Surgical Section, the seven characters are defined as follows:

Characters of ICD-10-PCS

1—Section of the ICD-10-PCS system where the code resides
2—The body system
3—Root operation (such as excision, resection
4—Specific body part
5—Approach used, such as percutaneous or open
6—Device left at the operative site such as indwelling catheter or pacemaker
7—Qualifier to provide additional information about the procedure (for example, to show if grafts are from the patient "autologous" or donor "nonautologous/allograft")

An example of an ICD-10-PCS code is 097F8DZ, Endoscopic dilation eustachian tube, right with intraluminal device:

0—Medical and Surgical Section
9—Body System—Ear, nose, sinus
7—Root operation is Dilation
F—Body Part is Eustachian tube, right
8—Via natural or artificial opening is Endoscopic
D—Device is Intraluminal
Z—No qualifier

To allow for complete coding using ICD-10-PCS, required documentation may be more than was required with ICD-9-CM. It is important that there must be a way that coders can communicate with the physicians to obtain any missing documentation to allow for consistent and timely coding using ICD-10-PCS. Some facilities use clinical documentation specialists to review documentation during the patient stay, so that ongoing communication about documentation needs is facilitated while the patient's medical chart is being completed.

Overview of ICD-9-CM

ICD-9-CM has been used in the United States for coding diagnoses and procedures since the 1970s. As it is replaced by ICD-10-CM and ICD-10-PCS, healthcare facilities will still have a need to continue to understand and utilize the ICD-9-CM coding system. Claims filed before the implementation date will need to be coded in ICD-9-CM. If any recovery audit contractor (RAC) or other audits are performed on older records, there must be someone who remains knowledgeable on ICD-9-CM to respond to audit results. Since data from codes are used by various reporting agencies and for reimbursement, careful interpretation of data and comparisons between the different coding systems should be done with caution.

ICD-9-CM is published in three volumes. Volume 1 is known as the Tabular List. It contains the numerical listing of codes that represent diseases and injuries. Volume 2 is the Alphabetic Index, which consists of an Alphabetic Index for all the codes listed in Volume 1. ICD-9-CM follows the same structure and patterns that are used in ICD-10-CM but is not as detailed as the ICD-10-CM system. The Tabular List and Alphabetic Index for Procedures are published as Volume 3 of ICD-9-CM, and this volume is used to report procedures performed on hospital inpatients. There is no procedure section in ICD-10-CM; hence, Volume 3 was replaced by ICD-10-PCS.

Other Issues in Coding Diagnoses

In many circumstances, the physician may not know the patient's diagnosis; hence, the coder may only be able to code the patient's signs and symptoms. It is important to understand the difference between coding signs and symptoms. A sign is visible evidence that the physician can determine objectively (for example, overactive bowel sounds and laceration to the skin). A symptom is a subjective, descriptive term, usually in the patient's own words, for example, "my head hurts."

Signs and symptoms must be coded with care. If a sign or symptom is a common occurrence with a particular diagnosis, it is not coded once the diagnosis has been made. If a sign or symptom occurs that is not a part of the normal disease process, that condition is coded.

In the emergency department setting, the physician may not be able to make an exact diagnosis and will recommend that the patient follow-up with his or her primary care physician. In these instances, the documentation may only substantiate coding of the patient's signs and symptoms. In the physician's office and outpatient or emergency department coding, the coding professional may only code the condition to the highest known cause. In these situations, conditions noted as "suspected," "rule out," or "possible" should not be coded.

This stipulation is not the same for hospital inpatient coding. In hospital inpatient coding, if the physician lists a condition as "suspected," "rule out," or "possible," the condition can be coded as if it exists. This is because inpatient stays are typically paid based on the resources needed to care for the patient. In these instances, sometimes the physician will want the signs and symptoms coded as well for use in further study. Official coding guidelines include rules on when signs and symptoms should be coded separately.

Laboratory reports usually show "normal" values, and when searching through the patient's record, the coder may find a value that is not within normal range. A slightly elevated potassium level may indicate Hyperkalemia E87.5 (an abnormally high concentration of potassium in the blood). However, the results may not be enough above normal limits to be considered significant. It is up to the physician to make this determination. The coding professional should query the physician and should not code hyperkalemia without clarification from the physician. Abnormal findings in the chart are coded only if the physician indicates that these findings have a clinical significance.

Medical Necessity

The Balanced Budget Act of 1997 requires that the physician must provide a diagnosis to substantiate the necessity of any test performed by another entity (hospital, laboratory, or other physician). The diagnosis or other medical information should include the reason for the test, which can be a sign, symptom, or diagnosis.

The term "medically necessary" typically has to do more with insurance coverage. Physicians may judge that a patient medically needs a procedure; however, many insurance companies, including Medicare, have rules that specify items that can be denied because of lack of medical necessity.

Medicare only allows coverage for services and items that are "medically reasonable and necessary" for the diagnosis and treatment of a patient. Medical necessity may be determined according to several factors including the following:

- Items or services provided to the patient must be appropriate for that patient's treatment or diagnosis.
- Documentation (when identified as required or when requested) supports the medical need.
- The frequency of service or dispensing of an item is within the accepted standards of medical practice.

Revisions to ICD-10

ICD-10-CM is updated each year with changes effective on October 1 of that year. All changes are published in the *Federal Register*, the publication used by the federal government to officially notify the public regarding changes in laws, rules, and regulations. These updates are typically found within the rules governing changes in the Inpatient Prospective Payment System (IPPS). ICD-10-CM diagnoses changes are available for review on the NCHS website and changes to ICD-10-PCS are found on the CMS website. These updates should be incorporated into existing systems prior to the October 1 deadline.

ICD-11

The WHO is currently working on an update to the ICD coding system, known as ICD-11. This revision is being developed to reflect changes in medicine and technology. Because healthcare evolves with technology, ICD-11 is being designed to be more user friendly with the electronic health record (EHR) environment. It is anticipated that the WHO will release the new version in 2015, but it will not be ready for use in the United States for several years after, because the US must modify the WHO update to reflect medical and technological issues specific to US coding needs.

ICD-11 will work with terminologies such as SNOMED CT and will have a more comprehensive approach to classifying morbidity and mortality. SNOMED CT is a widely used terminology designed for the EHR. It contains more than 300,000 concepts with specific definitions organized by a hierarchial system. SNOMED CT is being implemented in many software systems to provide detailed information and specific clinical information about the EHR. It is too specific to be used effectively as a reimbursement system, but it can be used in conjunction with coding systems, such as the ICD classification system.

Because there are multiple countries who have adapted ICD for use in their healthcare systems, ICD-11 is being configured for consistency among all users. Terms will be defined in greater detail to assure that their meanings are clearly identified, similar to how ICD-10-PCS has defined overlapping terms such as excision and resection.

Currently, a draft version of ICD-11 is available online to the public. Healthcare professionals who wish to become involved in the ICD-11 creation process can register on the WHO website to make comments and proposals for changes.

Even though the current process has been slow, healthcare workers in the US transitioning to ICD-10 should be encouraged by the updates being made in ICD-10. To ease future transition processes, while waiting for the ICD-11 system to become finalized, changes are being made in ICD-10 to reflect some of the topics and updates relating to new technology and information about the disease process that will be found in ICD-11.

Healthcare Common Procedure Coding System

HCPCS (pronounced "hick picks") is a collection of codes and descriptors used to represent healthcare procedures, supplies, products, and services. When the Medicare program was first implemented in the early 1980s, the Health Care Financing Administration (HCFA, now known as CMS) found it necessary to expand the HCPCS system because not all supplies, procedures, and services could be coded using the CPT system. An example of this shortcoming is durable medical equipment (DME). CPT does not contain codes for DME. Therefore, CMS developed an additional level of codes to report supplies and services that are not in CPT. CMS also made the determination that the CPT system did not provide enough specificity for coding procedures to allow for correct Medicare reimbursement.

Purpose and Use

In 1983, Medicare introduced HCPCS to promote uniform reporting and statistical data collection of medical procedures, supplies, products, and services. Most state Medicaid programs also used portions of the HCPCS coding system. Physicians and providers use HCPCS codes to report the services and procedures they deliver.

Overview of Structure

The structure of HCPCS is divided into two code levels or groups: I and II. Each are explained in detail, below.

Level I

Level I codes are the AMA's CPT codes. These five digit codes and two digit modifiers are copyrighted by the AMA. CPT codes primarily cover physicians' services but also are used for hospital outpatient coding. CPT codes are updated annually, effective January 1. If a CPT code description includes the term "specify," this should serve as a flag for coders to look for a more specific HCPCS national code. Sometimes Level I codes (CPT) are used in conjunction with Level II HCPCS codes, and in some instances either one or the other is used independently.

Level II

Level II codes, also called National Codes, are maintained by CMS. With the exception of temporary codes, Level II codes are updated annually on January 1.

Uses of Level II Codes

Level II codes were developed to code medical services, equipment, and supplies that are not included in CPT. There can be confusion regarding which codes are included in the HCPCS coding system. Level I codes are most often referred to merely as CPT. Technically, HCPCS includes both Level I (CPT) and Level II codes. The codes are alphanumeric and start with an alphabetic character from A to V. The alphabetic character is followed by four numeric characters. The alphabetic character identifies the code section and type of service or supply coded. These codes are often referred to by their alphabetic character, such as the codes that start with letter J are commonly known as "J codes" such as:

> **J1826 Injection, interferon beta-1a, 30 mcg**
> **J1835 Injection, itraconazole, 50 mg**

Temporary National Codes

Temporary codes begin with the letters G, K, or Q and are updated throughout the year. These codes are intended to meet, within a short time frame, the operational needs of a particular payer not addressed by a previously existing national code. For example, Medicare may need additional codes before the next scheduled annual HCPCS update to implement newly issued coverage policies or legislative requirements. Other payers may use the temporary codes established by Medicare. The HCPCS National Panel may decide to replace temporary codes with permanent codes. However, if permanent codes are not established, temporary codes may remain indefinitely. Whenever a permanent code is established by the National Panel to replace a temporary code, the temporary code is deleted and cross-referenced to the new permanent code.

At times, Level II codes were designed to reflect code assignment based on Medicare payment regulations. To illustrate, table 1.1 shows the different code choices for patients undergoing a colonoscopy based on their medical necessity. Table 1.2 provides a list of the major sections in Level II.

Table 1.1 CPT/HCPCS code choices for colonoscopy

Medical Necessity for Colonoscopy	Appropriate Code
Problem, such as bleeding or polyps	CPT codes 45378–45392
Colorectal cancer screening, patient does not meet Medicare definition of high risk	G0121
Colorectal cancer screening, patient meets definition of high risk	G0105

Source: HCPCS Level II.

Table 1.2 HCPCS Level II section titles

Section	Title
A0000–A0999	Transport Services Including Ambulance
A4000–A4899	Medical and Surgical Supplies
A9000–A9999	Administrative, Miscellaneous, and Investigational
B4000–B9999	Enteral and Parenteral Therapy
D0000–D9999	Dental Procedures
E0100–E9999	Durable Medical Equipment
G0000–G9999	Procedures/Professional Services (Temporary)
J0000–J8999	Drugs Other Than Chemotherapy
J9000–J9999	Chemotherapy Drugs
K0000–K9999	Orthotic Procedures
L5000–L9999	Prosthetic Procedures
M0000–M0009	Medical Services
P2000–P2999	Laboratory Tests
Q0000–Q9999	Temporary Codes
R0000–R5999	Domestic Radiology Services
S0009–S9999	Temporary National Codes
V0000–V2999	Vision Services
V5000–V5299	Hearing Services

Source: HCPCS Level II.

Table 1.3   Sample HCPCS Level II modifiers

Modifier	Meaning
AA	Anesthesia services performed personally by anesthesiologist
E1	Upper left eyelid
E2	Lower left eyelid
E3	Upper right eyelid
E4	Lower right eyelid
LT	Left side
RT	Right side

Source: HCPCS Level II.

Level II also contains modifiers that can be used with all levels of HCPCS codes, including CPT codes. The modifiers permit greater reporting specificity in reference to the main code. Sample level II modifiers appear in table 1.3.

Current Procedural Terminology

CPT is maintained by the AMA. It was designed as a comprehensive descriptive listing of terms and codes used to report diagnostic and therapeutic procedures and medical services. CPT differs from ICD-10-CM and ICD-10-PCS in that it is considered a nomenclature or "naming" system. This designation is significant in that typically only the most appropriate and descriptive term to describe a procedure is used. For example, many physicians will refer to the procedure of passing a scope into the bladder as a "cystoscopy." Technically, however, the physician must go through the urethra to access the bladder, so the correct term used in CPT is Cystourethroscopy. It is important that users of CPT have a strong background in medical terminology, anatomy, and physiology to be able to translate medical language used by the physician into the correct terminology used by the CPT system.

CPT has been commonly used in the physician's office for many years. It was not used in the hospital extensively until the 1980s when HCFA (now CMS) mandated its use for hospital outpatient billing as part of the HCPCS coding system. There have been several major updates to the system since the original edition was published in 1966; the fourth edition, *CPT-4*, is currently in use. Because the codes are changed substantially every year, however, the AMA dropped the "-4" and publishes the book with the year date; for example, the CPT book in 2013 is published as *CPT 2013*. CPT is updated annually by the AMA's CPT Editorial Panel. This panel is composed of physicians and other healthcare professionals who revise, modify, and update the publication.

The Editorial Panel gets advice on revisions from the CPT Advisory Committee. This committee is nominated by the AMA House of Delegates and is composed of representatives from more than 90 medical specialties and healthcare providers. As defined by the AMA, the committee has three objectives:

- Serve as a resource to the Editorial Panel by giving advice on procedure coding and nomenclature as relevant to the member's specialty
- Provide documentation to staff and the Editorial Panel regarding the medical appropriateness of various medical and surgical procedures
- Suggest revisions to CPT

Purpose and Use

The purpose of CPT is to provide a system for standard terminology and coding to report medical procedures and services. CPT is one of the most widely used systems for reporting medical services to health insurance carriers. In addition, it is used for other administrative purposes, such as developing guidelines for medical care review. Organizations that collect data for medical education and research purposes also use CPT.

CMS currently requires that CPT codes be used to report medical services provided to patients in specific settings. Starting in 1983, HCFA (now CMS) required that CPT be used to report services provided to Medicare Part B beneficiaries. In October 1986, HCFA required state Medicaid agencies to use CPT as part of the Medicaid Management Information System. As part of the Omnibus Budget Reconciliation Act, HCFA required in July 1987 that CPT be used for reporting outpatient hospital surgical procedures and ambulatory surgery center procedures. The most recent mandate for CPT use occurred with the final rule of HIPAA.

HIPAA mandates that CPT be used as the required code set for physicians' services and other medical services, such as physical therapy and most laboratory procedures.

Overview of Structure

The CPT code book consists of an introduction, eight sections containing the codes, appendices, and an index. Five digit codes are used throughout the CPT system, and most are numeric, although specific sections include an alphabetic character.

Sections

The sections are as follows:

Evaluation and Management	99210–99499
Anesthesia	00100–01999
Surgery	10040–69990
Radiology	70010–79999
Pathology and Laboratory	80049–89399
Medicine	90281–99602
Category II Codes	0001F–6005F
Category III Codes	0003T–0170T

Each of these sections begins with guidelines containing specific instructions and definitions that are unique to the section. Coding professionals must understand the information in the guidelines in order to code correctly from each section.

Introduction

The introduction contains a list of the code book section numbers, their sequences, and instructions for use. Information that appears in the introduction applies to all sections of the code book. A coder who is unfamiliar with CPT coding should read the introduction.

Symbols and punctuation marks are used to assist with correct usage of CPT codes. The symbols used in the CPT code book are explained in the introduction and are found at the bottom of each page of the coding section of the book.

Coding Conventions

There are several symbols and conventions used in the CPT book to alert the coding professional to use care in assigning the proper codes:

Symbol	Description
;	The semicolon is used in conjunction with indentations in the tabular section of the book to save space. The indented statements following another code description include part of the description in the preceding code.
▲	The triangle identifies procedures where the definition has changed substantially in the revised CPT book.
•	The bullet is used to identify procedures that have been added to the newest addition of the CPT book.
+	The plus symbol is used to show that the code is an "add-on" code and should never be used first or by itself.
#	The symbol for a resequenced code is the hashtag and indicates that the code is placed out of numeric sequence. This is done to allow placement of related procedures within the same family of codes when there is not an available code in that location.
o	Recycled or reinstated codes are indicated with the "o" symbol to identify codes that have been deleted that are being used again.
◎	The bull's-eye symbol is used to show that moderate/conscious sedation is included in the main procedure and is not coded separately.
Ø	The "don't" or null sign is found in front of codes that are exempt for the use of modifier 51.
> <	The facing triangles or "bowties" are used to identify new or revised text in the instruction and usage notes in CPT. Notes are used throughout the CPT book, so the coder should pay particular attention to any notes and follow the instructions carefully.

Category Codes

Beginning in the CPT 2002 book, references were made to "category codes." These are Category I, II, and III codes. Category I codes are the main CPT codes found in the largest section of the code book. Because it sometimes takes many years for new codes to be added to the code book, the AMA decided to develop other codes for testing and usage in the billing process. Category II codes were first published in the 2004 book, and according to CPT, they were designed as "supplemental tracking codes that can be used for performance measurement." Although these codes are optional, they can be used to provide greater specificity regarding a patient's visit and treatment details. All Category II codes end in the letter F, such as 2000F, blood pressure measured.

Category III codes were added to the CPT book to allow for temporary coding assignment for new technology and services that do not meet the rigorous requirements necessary to be added to the main section of the CPT book. Category III codes are alphanumeric (four numbers followed by the letter T) and their use is mandatory when applicable. Codes in the Category III section are evaluated and added every six months. As Category I codes (codes ranging from 00100 to 99499) are created to describe new procedures, the corresponding temporary category III codes will be deleted from the CPT system. Category II and Category III codes are found in the code book just behind the Medicine section. Insurance companies vary on their acceptance of these codes. An example of a Category III code is: 0210T Speech audiometry threshold, automated.

Appendices

Appendices follow the last section of codes. They provide information to help the coding professional in the coding process. Appendix A in the CPT code book provides a complete list of modifiers and their descriptions. Modifiers are written as two digit codes that follow the main CPT codes. For example, the two digit modifier for bilateral procedures services is modifier –50.

Another example of an important appendix in the CPT code book is appendix B. It includes a complete summary of the additions, deletions, and revisions that have been implemented for the current CPT edition. It can be used to update information and data that contain CPT codes. Any facility that uses preprinted forms such as encounter forms or fee tickets should review appendix B to cross reference any changes that require updating of the form.

Use of the Alphabetic Index

The Alphabetic Index is used to guide the coder to the appropriate code or range of codes. It is probably the point in the book that causes the most confusion because there are several different ways to look up a term. When locating a code in the alphabetical index, the coding professional should note if the code numbers are separated by commas or with a dash.

The CPT alphabetic index provides several different ways to help the coding professional locate a main term. **Main Terms** (listed in bold type in the index) may be found by searching under one of six categories:

- Procedure or Service—such as **Aspiration**
- Organ—such as **Kidney**
- Condition—such as **Tumor**
- Synonyms (another name for something)—such as **Renal—see Kidney**
- Eponyms (procedure named after a person)—such as **Mitchell Procedure**
- Abbreviations—such as **ADL—see Activities of Daily Living**

The most common way to locate a main term is by looking up the name of the procedure. Coding professionals begin their search for the correct CPT code by checking the alphabetic index in the above order until finding a likely code to describe the procedure performed. Main terms are followed by subterms. The subterms modify the main terms and are indented under them. The coding professional should then verify the code(s) selected in the main section of the code book to be certain the code best describes the procedure(s) performed. For example:

```
Abdomen
        Abdominal wall
        Debridement
                Infected            11005–11006
        Removal
                Mesh.               11008
                Prosthesis          11008
        Repair
                Hernia              49491–49496, 49501, 49507,
                                    49521, 49590
        Tumor
                Excision            22900-22903
                Radical Resection   22904–22905
```

Modifiers

Modifiers are used in CPT to change the description of the procedure in a predictable manner. Some reasons modifiers are used are as follows:

- Only part of a service was completed.
- A bilateral procedure was performed.

- A procedure was increased or reduced.
- An unusual event occurred.
- A service had both a professional and a technical component.

Modifiers can be added to the code by attaching a two digit modifier to the five digit CPT code. For example, Bilateral Repair of initial inguinal hernia, reducible, of a 35-year-old patient would be coded to 49505 with modifier 50. Different insurance carriers prefer various methods of using the modifiers. Medicare also accepts certain modifiers on claims for outpatient hospital services. Modifiers that can be used in the hospital setting are located in Appendix A in the CPT code book. However, in some instances, Medicare has published instructions for modifier usage that does not match the definitions in the CPT book. It is important to stay updated on current information published by Medicare to ensure correct interpretation and usage of the modifiers for use in Outpatient Prospective Payment System (OPPS) billing.

Evaluation and Management Coding

The Evaluation and Management (E/M) coding section is used to report services for physician medical visits such as office and hospital visits and consultations. These categories are further divided into subcategories and levels of service. This section has many rules and complex guidelines requiring extensive training for the physician office coders. E/M service codes are also required for payment in the hospital setting under the OPPS but the rules for usage are very different from those for physician professional services. It is important to remember that these codes were designed primarily for physician billing, and the rules in CPT do not always apply when being used by hospitals under OPPS. For example, critical care codes (99291–99292) include a list of procedures that are not separately billable when performed in association with a critical care visit. Medicare will pay facilities when these are performed. The physician will not be paid additionally for reading a chest x-ray, but the hospital will be paid separately for performing the x-ray.

E/M codes can be used by physicians or other qualified healthcare professionals. They can also be used in some instances to report services provided by hospitals or other healthcare facilities. For billing of professional services, E/M codes are assigned based on the documentation in the patient's medical record. There are three key components that comprise an E/M code: extent of patient history, extent of physical examination, and medical decision making. Within those three components, CPT recognizes distinct levels.

Extent of Patient History

The lowest level of patient history is Problem Focused, which includes the chief complaint and a brief history of present illness or condition.

The next level is Expanded Problem Focused. This level includes the items at a condition or problem focused level plus a system review based on the patient's identified complaint.

To meet the documentation requirements for a detailed history, the physician or qualified healthcare professional has to document the chief complaint, an extended history of present illness, a symptom-pertinent system review extended to include a review of a limited number of additional systems, as well as pertinent past, family, and/or social history directly related to the patient's symptoms.

Comprehensive is the highest level of history. This includes documentation of the patient's chief complaint, extended history of present illness, a review of systems directly related to the symptom(s) identified in the history of the present illness, plus a review of all additional body systems. It also includes documentation of a complete past, family, and social history.

Extent of Examination

The second of the three key elements involves documentation of the physical examination. Like the history component, there are also four distinct levels of documentation required for correct coding. The lowest level of examination is Problem Focused, which involves an examination that is limited to the affected body area or organ system. Expanded Problem Focused is the next higher level. This would entail documentation showing an examination of the affected body area or organ system as well as other symptomatic or related organ systems. A Detailed Examination includes an extended examination of the affected body area(s) and other symptomatic or related organ system(s). The highest level is Comprehensive, which includes a general multisystem examination or a complete examination of a single organ system.

Medical Decision Making

The third key component in coding an E/M code is perhaps the most difficult of the three areas to document. This component takes into account the physician or qualified healthcare professional's knowledge and thought process required to establish a diagnosis and select a management option based on three areas. These three areas include the number of possible diagnoses or management options, the amount of data to be reviewed, and the risk of complications to the patient.

99212, Office or other outpatient visit for the evaluation and management of an established patient, requires at least two of the three key components:

- A problem-focused history
- A problem-focused examination
- Straightforward medical decision making

Counseling or coordination of care with other providers or agencies is provided consistent with the nature of the problem(s) and the patient's or family's needs. Usually, the presenting problem(s) are self-limited or minor. Typically, 10 minutes is spent face-to-face with the patient or family.

In addition to the three components listed in the previous section (extent of patient history, physical examination and medical decision making), other components that contribute to the patient's level of care include the following:

- Nature of presenting problem: the reason for the visit. This may be a symptom, disease, illness, or complaint.
- Counseling includes discussion with the patient and/or family concerning results of testing, treatment options, instructions for medication and follow-up, and education.
- Coordination of Care includes coordination and communication with other healthcare personnel regarding treatment and further care of the patient.

Time can be an overriding factor in some categories if the physician or qualified healthcare professional documents that more than half of the visit was spent counseling the patient. To get credit for time, the physician or qualified healthcare professional must document the total time of the visit as well as the total amount of time spent counseling the patient. This is physician counseling time, not time spent by a nurse, dietitian, or other ancillary provider.

New Versus Established Patient

Some of the categories of patients are divided according to whether the patient is new or established. A patient who has not previously seen a physician or qualified healthcare professional, or a physician or qualified healthcare professional of the same specialty in the same practice within three years is considered a new patient.

Documentation Guidelines

CMS has established documentation guidelines to promote uniformity in evaluation and management services coding. There are two published sets of guidelines; the first was published in 1995, and the second in 1997. The main difference in these two sets is found in the examination area. Typically, specialists fare better with the 1997 guidelines because they get credit for more documentation of bulleted items within fewer body systems. General practitioners such as family practice or internal medicine tend to do better under the 1995 guidelines because they receive credit for review of more body systems, even though the documentation might not be as detailed as described by a specialist. CMS has made several attempts to create one set of coding guidelines, but until that happens, the physician or qualified healthcare professional must use either the 1995 or 1997 guidelines, whichever is more advantageous. These guidelines are found on the CMS website and many vendors sell both documentation and audit tools to use in ensuring correct usage of the codes.

Other E/M Coding Notes

Generally, only one E/M code per physician or qualified healthcare professional per patient per day is assigned. If the physician or qualified healthcare professional sees the patient more than one time on the same day, the coding professional should assign only the highest level of visit for that calendar day as the physician or qualified healthcare professional builds on documentation and knowledge of the patient's condition throughout the various levels of care during that day. There are exceptions to this rule, such as a patient discharged from one facility and admitted to another on the same date of service.

Just as in assignment of diagnosis codes, coding with CPT should be done only through careful review of the documentation available. Figure 1.1 illustrates the rules that coders must follow when assigning codes to procedures that are performed:

Figure 1.1 Rules for CPT Coding

1. Analyze the information given by the physician or qualified healthcare professional to determine the service that was performed.
2. Locate the main term in the Alphabetic Index.
3. Select the appropriate subterm(s) listed below the main term.
4. Note the code number(s) located next to the subterm selected.
   - If a single code number is given, locate the code in the numerical section of CPT. Verify the code and match the description to the procedural statement.
   - If two or more codes are given, separated by a comma, or if a range of codes is given, locate each of these codes in the index and select the most appropriate code(s).
5. Never code directly from the Alphabetic Index.
6. Read all notes that pertain to the code number selected. These notes may appear at the beginning of a section, subsection or appear under the code description.
7. Select the appropriate modifier if needed.
8. Code all components of the service, following the instructions in the CPT book.

Chapter 2

Reimbursement Overview

Medicare

Medicare was initially designed in the 1960s to provide catastrophic medical coverage for older Americans who had paid into the Social Security system through their employers. It was not designed to be the full coverage insurance plan that it has become. It has changed over the years to include other individuals such as those with disabilities and those with end-stage renal disease (ESRD). Moreover, Medicare has been modified by Congress to include more preventive care such as cancer screening.

The federal agency that oversees the Medicare program is the Centers for Medicare and Medicaid Services (CMS). According to CMS, "a more modern Medicare brings more affordable health care, prescription drug coverage to all people with Medicare, expanded health plan choices, improved healthcare access for rural Americans, and preventive care services, such as flu shots and mammograms."

Medicare enrollees are known as beneficiaries. Beneficiaries are typically patients older than 65 years, but others may qualify for Medicare benefits, such as the disabled, specified in the Social Security Act. Medicare is divided into four main parts (Medicare Parts A through D), each covering different services.

Medicare contracts with local insurance companies to provide services for Medicare beneficiaries in the region. These contractors manage the Medicare program for a specific geographic region of the country and must follow national coverage determinations (NCDs) as set forth by Medicare. They also can establish local policies for items not addressed in the federal guidelines. In the past, the contractors who paid the bills for hospital services (Part A claims) were known as the fiscal intermediary (FI) and the physician bills (Part B claims) were paid by the carrier. FIs and carriers have been replaced by the regional Medicare Administrative Contractors (MACs) who are responsible for both Part A and B Medicare. Corporate hospitals and groups that have facilities in multiple regions of the United States all may be assigned to the same contractor. The contractors may issue local coverage determinations (LCDs), formerly known as local medical review policies (LMRPs), which document a decision by the contractor (A/B MAC) whether to cover a particular service. These administrative and educational tools assist providers, physicians, and suppliers in submitting correct claims for payment and typically include information regarding diagnoses that validate medical necessity.

Medicare Part A

Medicare Part A pays for inpatient hospitalization and some skilled aftercare services, such as nursing home, home health, and hospice care for covered beneficiaries. Medicare patients have maximum benefit periods of 60 full days plus 30 days of coinsurance coverage. This benefit is renewable after the patient has not been in a hospital or skilled nursing facility for 60 days. Patients also have a lifetime reserve benefit of 60 additional days. Moreover, Medicare patients have a lifetime maximum of 190 inpatient psychiatric days of coverage.

Medicare Part B

Medicare Part B is designed to pay for physician-related services, some outpatient hospital services, durable medical equipment (DME), and supplies. Medicare beneficiaries must pay an additional monthly premium for this coverage. Certain services normally covered under Part A can be paid under Part B claims when patients have exhausted their Part A benefits.

DME such as wheelchairs, crutches, and other supplies are covered under the jurisdiction of a durable medical equipment regional carrier (DMERC). There are currently four regional carriers for DME, located in Chicago, Philadelphia, Dallas, and Denver. The DMERCs have a different set of rules and regulations than the area Medicare carrier. When a hospital provides DME services, it must be certified as a medical equipment provider and must follow special billing rules and regulations as set forth by Medicare and maintained by the regional DMERC.

Medicare Part C

Medicare Part C, or Medicare Advantage (MA), is a preferred provider organization (PPO) type of coverage for Medicare beneficiaries that offers options such as regional PPOs and specialized health plans for certain diagnoses. Medicare uses a statistical model to review the costs incurred for the enrollees to determine predictions for future years' healthcare expenses. This model is known as the principal inpatient diagnostic cost group (PIP-DCG) algorithm, a model designed to calculate each beneficiary's relative risk in terms of overall Medicare expenditures.

Medicare Part D

Medicare Part D represents the Medicare Prescription Drug Plan that provides assistance to Medicare beneficiaries who incur substantial drug expenses. The plan is voluntary and administered by various contractors. The beneficiary is responsible for an annual deductible and copayments, and Medicare reimburses a percentage of drug costs above established thresholds. During the first years of the plan, patients earning lower incomes were eligible for prescription drug benefits, but eventually all Medicare patients who are eligible for Medicare Part A or have Part B coverage also will be eligible for the Medicare prescription drug benefits. Beneficiaries have the following two options for receiving these benefits:

- Patients who choose to remain in the traditional Medicare coverage plans will have the option of joining a prescription drug plan (PDP) to obtain drug benefits for an additional charge.
- Patients can switch over to the Medicare Advantage plan and obtain hospital, physician, and prescription drug benefits from one company. The plan that includes medication coverage is known as Medicare Advantage-Prescription Drug (MA-PD).

The Medicare Prospective Payment System

As recently as the 1980s, the following scenario was not uncommon: A family member (for example, Grandma) was bedridden and living at home. When the family wanted to go on vacation, they left Grandma at the hospital for what was commonly referred to as respite care. Because of the lack of regulations surrounding Medicare payment, this type of scenario occurred even when there was no acute medical condition that would necessitate Grandma being treated in an acute care facility.

When Medicare was first developed, it paid claims to hospitals based on the fee-for-service reimbursement plan. The patient was admitted to the hospital where tests and other procedures were performed based on physician orders. After the patient went home, the hospital submitted a bill to Medicare, which paid based on a percentage of the total charges.

This type of indemnity plan actually served to reward physicians and hospitals for overutilization of services. Basically, when the doctor ordered a test, it was performed and Medicare paid the bill with little or no review of the appropriateness or the need for the services rendered. After a few years of this type of payment system, it became clear that the Medicare system was in jeopardy of running out of funding. The government soon realized that the Medicare program would not survive unless changes were made to the system. Consequently, the government started searching for ways to maintain better control over the system. It was at this time that the concept of a prospective payment system (PPS) was first discussed.

The family in the scenario above currently would have multiple options for taking care of Grandma, but if she did not meet criteria that justified an acute care admission, she would not be placed in the hospital for respite care. Currently, both Medicare and most insurance companies require a thorough preadmission assessment to allow patients to be cared for in the setting most appropriate for their conditions.

Characteristics of a PPS

Several key components characterize a system based on prospectively set prices, including the following:

- Payment rates are established in advance and fixed for the fiscal period to which they apply.
- Payment rates are not automatically determined by the hospital's past or current actual cost.
- Rates represent full payment for services provided.
- The hospital retains the profit or absorbs the loss of payment resulting from the difference between the rate of payment and the hospital's cost of caring for the patient.

Typically, the fiscal period mentioned above refers to the US government's fiscal year, which runs from October 1 to September 30. However, some of the newer payment systems are set up on other fiscal years, such as July 1 through June 30. At times, because of errors or changes in technology, some modifications are made to the payment systems quarterly or as needed throughout the year.

Under the PPS reimbursement system, there is a strong incentive for the facility to provide high quality care at the lowest possible cost. There has been an increase in the use of utilization review (UR) professionals and case managers to review the charts during the hospital encounter to ensure that the patient's care is being managed effectively. Prospective payment monitoring also has helped facilities to ensure that services provided are necessary for the patient at the acute level of care.

Because of many legislative changes in the Medicare system over the past 20 years, most types of Medicare services now are paid for under some sort of prospective payment methodology. PPSs exist today in almost all healthcare settings, including the following:

- Inpatient acute care hospitals
- Outpatient hospitals
- Physician offices
- Skilled nursing facilities
- Long-term care hospitals
- Home healthcare settings
- Inpatient rehabilitation facilities
- Inpatient psychiatric facilities

Structure and Organization of the Medicare Inpatient Acute Care PPS

The Social Security Act, as amended in 1982 by the Tax Equity and Fiscal Responsibility Act (TEFRA), mandated the use of a PPS for inpatient hospital services provided under Part A of Medicare. In the 1970s, a research team at Yale University classified patients into categories based on the diagnoses that caused them to be admitted to the hospital in order to determine why patients with similar cases differed in their usage of resources. Patients were divided into various categories that were medically meaningful so that all patients in the same category would be expected to respond in a clinically similar manner. The data were averaged statistically to show that patients placed in these categories used approximately equal amounts of the hospital's facilities and resources. The categories became known as diagnosis-related groups (DRGs). The DRG payment system, which has been in place since the 1980s, is used by Medicare to pay for hospital inpatient admissions. The latest revision, Medicare Severity-adjusted Diagnosis-Related Groups (MS-DRGs), has been designed to account for variations in severity of acutely ill patients and was implemented in 2007.

DRGs are derived from all the diagnoses and procedures listed in the *International Classification of Diseases, Ninth Revision, Clinical Modification (ICD-9-CM)* classification system. Medicare will transition the system to include ICD-10-CM and ICD-10-PCS codes when the new coding systems are implemented in 2014. DRGs are numbers signifying into which category the patient best fits. Grouping patients into categories that consume similar amounts of resources reveals typical and atypical patterns of utilization. The researchers who developed the DRG system were trying to define expected lengths of patient stays so that UR activities could be focused on atypical patients. Their design was not established with the intent for use as the basis for a payment system. However, when the government learned of the study, it became interested and funded a project in New Jersey to determine if this type of system would work as a reimbursement system.

From 1983 to 2007, hospitals subject to the Inpatient PPS were paid a specific amount for each discharge based on the DRG category in which the case was grouped. The DRG assignment is based on the patient's principal diagnosis, secondary diagnoses, procedures performed, and in some cases, age, sex, and discharge disposition. In fiscal year 2008, CMS updated the DRG system to include the division of secondary diagnoses into further categories to more accurately reflect the patient's severity of illness, or, the MS-DRG system.

Principal Diagnosis

The principal diagnosis is defined in the Uniform Hospital Discharge Data Set (UHDDS) as "that condition established, after study, to be chiefly responsible for occasioning the admission of the patient to the hospital for care" (NCHS 2013). This explanation helps to establish a standard definition when comparing data from different facilities but causes much confusion in coding. For example, if a patient is admitted with chest pain, and after testing, it is determined that the patient has an acute myocardial infarction (MI), the MI qualifies as the principal diagnosis. However, if the patient is admitted for the treatment of benign prostate hypertrophy and then after admission has a massive heart attack, even though the focus of the admission has changed, the principal diagnosis is the prostate condition with the heart attack counting as a complication.

Secondary Diagnoses

According to the UHDDS, secondary diagnoses include all conditions that "coexist at the time of admission, or develop subsequently, which affect the treatment received and/or the length of stay. Diagnoses that refer to an earlier episode, that have no bearing on the current hospital or nursing home stay, are to be excluded. Conditions should be coded that affect patient care in terms of requiring clinical evaluation; therapeutic treatment; diagnostic procedures; extended length of hospital or nursing home stay; or increased nursing care and/ or monitoring" (NCHS 2013). Secondary diagnoses may help to determine the grouping if they qualify as a complication or comorbidity (CC). Statistically, a CC is a "condition, which because of its presence with a specific principal diagnosis, would cause an increase in the length of stay by at least one day in at least 75 percent of the patients" (NCHS 2013). Complications are those conditions that arise after admission. If a patient is admitted with pneumonia and then has a stroke on the second day of hospitalization, the stroke would be considered a complication according to the UHDDS definition. This definition may not be the same as a complication due to, or caused by, a surgical or medical procedure.

A comorbidity is a condition that is present on admission, for example, a systemic disease such as type II diabetes, essential hypertension, or a concomitant acute illness or injury. These illnesses may cause a patient to recover at a slower rate than a patient without any additional complications. Through fiscal year 2007, with paired DRGs, a single CC has caused the patient's case to be grouped into the higher-weighted DRG. In the MS-DRG systems, some secondary diagnoses qualify as complications/comorbidities (CCs), or major complications/comorbidities (MCCs), because they greatly impact the resources needed to care for the patient. In many cases, the presence of a secondary condition that qualifies as an MCC will have a greater impact on the DRG weight and payment. For example:

MS-DRG 177   Respiratory Infections and Inflammations with MCC
Weight 2.0653

MS-DRG 178   Respiratory Infections and Inflammation with CC
Weight 1.4653

MS-DRG 179   Respiratory Infections and Inflammations without
CC/MCC   Weight 1.0025

Over the years, because of changes in medicine and the shift of care toward outpatient services, patients who were admitted to the hospital were more likely to have secondary conditions that were grouped into the CC category. Studies of 2006 data revealed that nearly 80 percent of patients had at least one secondary diagnosis that counted as a CC. As a result, the CC list no longer could be used as a mechanism for determining increased hospital resource usage. Medicare dramatically reduced the number of codes that counted as a CC in fiscal year 2008, with the intent that this change would decrease the number of patients having a CC in half.

CC/MCC Exclusion List

Medicare also developed a list of CC/MCC exclusions. Some secondary diagnoses may act as CCs or MCCs with certain diagnoses, but not with others. As such, those secondary conditions do not cause an increase in the amount of resources needed to care for the patient.

DRG Relative Weight

Each DRG is assigned a relative weight that represents the average resources required to care for a patient assigned to a specific DRG in relation to the national average of resources used to treat all Medicare cases. When DRG groups were first developed, there needed to be a way to compare the different groups according to the amount of resources utilized. To obtain a starting point for comparison, the average cost of all Medicare patients was established and assigned a relative weight of 1.0000. All patient cases were then divided into DRGs and ranked according to the number of resources utilized. As all other DRGs were compared with the average, they were assigned weights appropriate for their average resources used by patients in that group. For example, if one DRG uses twice as many resources as the average, it would be weighted at 2.0000. Conversely, if a group uses half as many resources as average, it would be weighted at 0.5000. Weights for all DRGs are updated every year and published in the *Federal Register*, with the changes becoming effective on October 1 of each year.

Each facility is assigned a base rate that takes into account various factors that have an impact on cost to care for patients in their area. These factors include the following:

- A wage index, which reflects that labor costs vary in different areas of the country
- Additional payments for those hospitals with treatment patterns that fall into specific categories such as:
  o A large share of low income or indigent patients
  o Teaching hospitals to reflect the higher cost of providing medical education

The base rate is then multiplied by the DRG weight to determine the actual payment rate for that facility.

Outliers

When the patient's costs exceed a predetermined cost threshold, the facility may be eligible to receive additional reimbursement added to the DRG base rate. This patient is known as a cost outlier. If the patient qualifies as an outlier, a determination of additional payment is made, which begins at the cost threshold amount. The hospital's cost-to-charge ratios are used to determine whether a patient's costs are greater than the threshold amount. After the threshold limit is reached, the hospital receives a percentage of costs above this amount.

Post-Acute Care Transfer Policy

Hospitals must carefully report the patient's discharge status on the billing form because it can have an impact on reimbursement. This is true even of a patient who is transferred from the acute care setting to the another unit within the hospital, such as a long-term care, swing bed service, or is discharged to home with orders for home health services to continue the patient's treatment or care.

Because the DRG payment is supposed to pay for all care associated with diagnoses and treatment necessary to care for a patient, when a patient is transferred before completion of that care, the rate of DRG payment is adjusted to account for the change. For example, when a patient is transferred from one facility that is paid under the inpatient PPS (IPPS) to another facility also paid under the IPPS system, the two facilities share the DRG total payment. During the past several years, Medicare has developed a post-acute care transfer policy that also adjusts the DRG payment based on incomplete care. According to CMS.gov, DRG payments are reduced when:

> The beneficiary's length of stay (LOS) is at least one day less than the geometric mean LOS for the DRG; the beneficiary is transferred to an another hospital covered by the Acute Care Hospital IPPS or, for certain MS-DRGs, discharged to a post-acute setting; the beneficiary is transferred to a hospital that does not have an agreement to participate in the Medicare Program (effective October 1, 2010); and, the beneficiary is transferred to a CAH [critical access hospital] (effective October 1, 2010). The following post-acute care settings are included in the transfer policy:
>> Long-term care hospitals;
>> Rehabilitation facilities;
>> Psychiatric facilities;
>> SNFs;
>> Home Healthcare when the beneficiary receives clinically related care that begins within 3 days after the hospital stay;
>> Rehabilitation distinct part (DP) units located in an acute care hospital or a CAH;
>> Psychiatric DP units located in an acute care hospital or a CAH;
>> Cancer hospitals; and
>> Children's hospitals.

Grouper Software

CMS established the grouper program, which is an automated classification system that uses the prescribed information to assign discharges to their proper DRGs. The MAC, or organization processing hospital inpatient claims for CMS, assigns the proper DRG using the grouper program. Most hospitals assign DRGs for all cases to facilitate quality management activities and estimate revenue, but it is the DRG assigned by the MAC's group that determines final reimbursement.

Annual Updates

The IPPS system was designed to be modified once each year to allow for updates. The largest update occurs because of the creation, revision, or deletion of ICD-9-CM and the ICD-10-CM and ICD-10-PCS codes as these new systems are implemented. Also, because the IPPS system is based on statistical and medical cohesiveness, there are times when changes need to be made, such as a redistribution of codes to different DRG groupings. These changes are published in the *Federal Register* with an effective date of October 1 of each year. The ICD-10-CM and ICD-10-PCS coding systems may be updated twice per year (October and April) to allow for the addition of codes for new technology. When new codes are added midyear, they are assigned to current DRG groups until the following October, when the DRG groups are updated, as needed.

Severity of Illness

One common criticism of the Medicare DRG system is that the severity of a patient's disease is not always directly reflected in the DRG assignment. With paired DRGs, the presence of a single CC has been shown to significantly add to the resources needed to fully treat the patient. Therefore, patients within one DRG group may vary greatly in the number of additional diagnoses they have, meaning that patients in the same DRG could consume quite different quantities of resources. This is supposed to be accounted for in the law of averages, as one patient may use fewer resources for his or her care and one may use more; hence, theoretically the hospital breaks even. In response to the concerns of the DRG system not capturing of illness (SOI) data, CMS researched several variations to the DRG system and made the decision to replace DRG's with MS-DRGs.

Medicare Severity-Adjusted DRG

Beginning in fiscal year 2008, Medicare implemented a large-scale update to the DRG system to allow for more appropriate payment for patients with higher SOI. This update is known as the MS-DRG system. The classification groups are divided based on the presence of secondary diagnoses that have been separated into three different categories: major CC, CC, and non-CC. A major CC includes those conditions that have a consistent major impact on the resources needed to care for a patient and include acute exacerbation of significant chronic illnesses, advanced or end stage chronic illnesses, significant acute diseases, such as MI, acute renal failure, cerebrovascular accident, and chronic diseases associated with extensive debility. CCs are those secondary conditions that have an impact on resource usage, such as left heart failure, and non-CCs are secondary conditions that do not significantly impact SOI or resource usage, such as chronic obstructive pulmonary disease (COPD) or congestive heart failure.

Hospital-Acquired Conditions

As part of Medicare's "pay for performance" policies, hospitals are no longer rewarded with higher reimbursement for conditions that could have been prevented. In order to capture this information, since 2007, hospitals have been required to indicate whether or not each patient's medical condition was "present on admission" (POA). If the hospital-acquired condition (HAC) list was present on the patient's admission, Medicare will continue to assign the patient's discharge to a higher paying MS-DRG. If a patient acquires a condition that is on the HAC list after admission (not POA), it will be grouped into an MS-DRG as if that condition was not present. For example, if a patient was admitted with a secondary condition of a Stage III pressure ulcer, this would count as a CC and the patient's case would be grouped into a higher weighted MS-DRG. However, if this condition occurred after admission, then the hospital would be paid as though the pressure ulcer did not exist because this should have been a preventable condition.

Case-Mix Index

The case-mix index for a hospital is defined as the average MS-DRG weight for all patients over a specified time period. A high case-mix index would signify that the patients treated in the facility were, on average, sicker than those in facilities with a lower case-mix index.

Other Uses of MS-DRGs

Although MS-DRGs are primarily used for payment, the hospital can use the data for many other purposes, such as UR. By examining the MS-DRG data, the facility can examine utilization patterns among similar groups of patients to study variances and identify areas for improvement. Hospitals can review differences among physicians to determine reasons for variations in practice patterns or overutilization of ancillary services. Reports can be generated, such as the top 10 medical and surgical MS-DRGs, which can provide data, can be reviewed to determine appropriateness of services or provide topics for auditing.

Financial services can use the data for hospital cost analysis with up to date information on MS-DRGs for patients being discharged and the costs for treating these patients. The revenue can be monitored in a timely manner to detect patterns of high cost/low reimbursement. Additionally, the data can be used to help plan for new services, such as determining whether the facility should expand certain services. Moreover, they can be used for benchmarking best practices with other, similar facilities for epidemiology studies and research.

Each year, as the system is updated, an attempt is made to accurately reflect appropriate payment necessary to treat the changing Medicare population. As Medicare continues to research variations and alternatives to the IPPS system, healthcare professionals should monitor these changes and their impact on reimbursement and case-mix index.

Other Medicare Inpatient PPSs

Because the federal government considered MS-DRGs to be so successful in managing costs and resource consumption in the acute care hospital inpatient setting, legislation has been passed that requires prospective payment-type systems in other healthcare settings. In this section, some of the Medicare systems in place for reimbursement in settings other than acute care hospitals are discussed.

Long-Term Acute Care PPS

The Balanced Budget Refinement Act of 1999 and the Benefits Improvement and Protection Act of 2000 established the requirements for a PPS for long-term acute care hospitals (LTCHs), effective with discharges on or after October 1, 2002. Medicare defines LTCHs as hospitals that:

> Have an average inpatient length of stay greater than 25 days. These hospitals typically provide extended medical and rehabilitative care for patients who are clinically complex and may suffer from multiple acute or chronic conditions. Services may include comprehensive rehabilitation, respiratory therapy, cancer treatment, head trauma treatment, and pain management (Hull 2003).

The Medicare severity-adjusted long-term care hospital prospective payment system (MS-LTCH-PPS) is based on the IPPS system with modifications made to account for differences in the long-term care patient. There are also special rules covering occurrences such as short stays, very high cost admissions, and interrupted stays. This system was put into place in October 2003. Patients' stays are grouped into MS-LTC-DRG categories based on their diagnoses, procedures performed, age, gender, and discharge status. Like the inpatient MS-DRG system, CMS specifies that the MS-LTC-DRG grouping reflects "the typical resources used for treating such a patient." Also like the MS-DRG System, the MS-LTC-DRG system was designed to pay only one amount of reimbursement per hospitalization, which is assigned at discharge.

Coding professionals must follow the same rules as those used for coding IPPS, which includes following official coding guidelines and the UHDDS definitions. This includes the definition for principal diagnosis, complications, comorbidities, conditions that affect treatment, and all procedures performed during MS-LTC-DRG as is used for inpatient MS-DRG grouping. The payment rates are based on the data in the Medicare Provider Analysis and Review (MedPAR) database consisting of claims previously submitted by LTC hospitals.

Inpatient Rehabilitation Hospital PPS

Implementation of a per discharge PPS for inpatient rehabilitation facilities (IRFs) was authorized in Section 4421 of the Balanced Budget Act of 1997 (Public Law 105-33), as amended by Section 125 of the Medicare, Medicaid, and State Children's Health Insurance Program (SCHIP) Balanced Budget Refinement Act of 1999 (Public Law 106-113), and by Section 305 of the Medicare, Medicaid, and SCHIP Benefits Improvement and Protection Act of 2000 (Public Law 106-554), authorized through a new Section 1886(j) of the Social Security Act.

In 1995, CMS sponsored a study by Rand Corporation to develop an IRF per discharge PPS using a system known as functional independence measures–functional-related groups (FIM-FRGs). This study was updated in 1999 to reflect payment information, including facility payment adjustments and the impact of other diagnoses (comorbidities) on patient resource utilization.

To account for the types of patients treated in IRFs, this system uses information from the patient assessment instrument (PAI). The information from the resulting IRF patient assessment instrument (IRF-PAI) is entered electronically into grouper software, which determines the health insurance prospective payment system (HIPPS) codes used to establish reimbursement. The software is known as Inpatient Rehabilitation Validation and Entry (IRVEN). The HIPPS codes are then grouped into one of 100 case-mix groups, which determine reimbursement for the hospitalization.

Inpatient Psychiatric Facilities

The Balanced Budget Refinement Act of 1999 required that a PPS be established for licensed inpatient psychiatric hospitals and hospital-based psychiatric units. This inpatient psychiatric facility (IPF) PPS was phased in over a three year period starting with discharges on or after January 1, 2005. Like the other PPS systems, this system is based on the inpatient DRG system with modifications to account for differences unique to the patients needing intensive psychiatric treatment.

Ambulatory Payment Classifications (APCs): Medicare Outpatient PPS

As the IPPS system was used on a regular basis, facilities shifted patients to the outpatient setting, which meant that outpatient costs increased dramatically and laws were passed that mandated the creation of a PPS-type payment methodology for outpatient services. In August 2000, Medicare implemented a PPS for outpatient hospital services. The Outpatient PPS, better known as OPPS, is similar in many ways to the IPPS system established in the 1980s. The OPPS is a classification system that helps to explain the types and amounts of resources an outpatient visit requires. It was devised to help control costs and improve efficiency in the delivery of outpatient care through changes in facility management, communications, and cost accounting and planning. Reimbursement is made by grouping patient services into a system known as ambulatory payment classification, or APCs. Healthcare facilities have been required to reevaluate their outpatient coding, billing, and documentation processes and adjust to this major source of change.

Grouping Codes in the APC System

The APC system is based on code descriptions provided by the HCPCS/CPT coding system. Like the MS-DRG system, procedures and services within APCs are grouped according to five different criteria. These include resource homogeneity, which means that resources are fairly constant across the services included in the group; and clinical homogeneity, which groups codes together that are of the same organ or etiology, same degree of extensiveness, or utilize the same method of treatment.

When setting up the APC system, criteria were used to account for lower volume procedures including provider concentration, a term used to signify that the service is provided in a limited number of hospitals; hence, the impact of the payment for that service is high. Another is known as Frequency of Service. In other words, separate groups were not created for services performed infrequently unless a provider concentration was found. The last criterion was that of minimal opportunities for upcoding and code fragmentation, which means that the groups are both broad and inclusive to discourage using a code in a higher paying group without documentation to support the code usage.

Status Indicators

Medicare assigned an alphabetical character to each HCPCS code to indicate the payment methodology utilized for reimbursement. These alphabetical characters are known as status indicators. For example, some items normally encountered in the outpatient department, such as laboratory procedures, are paid on a set fee schedule and are therefore not included in payment under the OPPS rules. Those CPT codes used to describe the laboratory test would have an "A" status indicator. See table 2.1 for a sample list of outpatient PPS status indicators.

Packaging

APCs were created to include payment for all supplies, procedures, and services that are commonly performed as part of the overall payment rate. For example, most cataract surgeries include removing the damaged lens and replacing it with a new artificial lens; therefore, most cataract procedures include the cost of the lens supply within the payment that the facility will receive for the procedure of cataract removal. Supplies such as surgical dressings are packaged into the APC payment rate for the procedure with which it is associated. Codes for packaged items have a Status Indicator of "N."

Examples of packaged items include the use of the operating/treatment/procedure room, observation bed, anesthesia, medical and surgical supplies and equipment, surgical dressings, supplies, and equipment for administering and monitoring anesthesia or sedation, drugs, pharmaceutical and biologic agents (unless they meet the standards for additional payments for expensive drugs such as chemotherapy agents).

Table 2.1   Status indicators

Indicator	Item/Code/Service	OPPS Payment Status
A	Services furnished to a hospital outpatient that are paid under a fee schedule or payment system other than OPPS, for example: • Ambulance services • Clinical diagnostic laboratory services • Nonimplantable prosthetic and orthotic devices • EPO for ESRD patients • Physical, occupational, and speech therapy • Routine dialysis services for ESRD patients provided in a certified dialysis unit of a hospital • Diagnostic mammography • Screening mammography	Not paid under OPPS. Paid by fiscal intermediaries under a fee schedule or payment system other than OPPS.
B	Codes that are not recognized by OPPS when submitted on an outpatient hospital Part B bill type (12x and 13x).	Not paid under OPPS. • May be paid by intermediaries when submitted on a different bill type, for example, 75x (CORF), but not paid under OPPS. • An alternate code that is recognized by OPPS when submitted on an outpatient hospital Part B bill type (12x and 13x) may be available.

(Continued)

Table 2.1 Status indicators (*continued*)

Indicator	Item/Code/Service	OPPS Payment Status
C	Inpatient procedures	Not paid under OPPS. Admit patient. Bill as inpatient.
D	Discontinued codes	Not paid under OPPS or any other Medicare payment system.
E	Items, codes, and services: 1. That are not covered by Medicare based on statutory exclusion. 2. That are not covered by Medicare for reasons other than statutory exclusion. 3. That are not recognized by Medicare but for which an alternate code for the same item or service may be available. 4. For which separate payment is not provided by Medicare.	Not paid under OPPS or any other Medicare payment system.
F	Corneal tissue acquisition; Certain CRNA services and Hepatitis B vaccines	Not paid under OPPS. Paid at reasonable cost.
G	Pass through drugs and biologicals	Paid under OPPS; Separate APC payment includes pass through amount.
H	Pass through device categories	Separate cost-based pass through payment; Not subject to coinsurance.

Indicator	Item/Code/Service	OPPS Payment Status
K	1. Non-Pass through drugs and biologicals 2. Therapeutic radiopharmaceuticals 3. Brachytherapy sources 4. Blood and blood products	1. Paid under OPPS; Separate APC payment. 2. Paid under OPPS; Separate APC payment. 3. Paid under OPPS; Separate APC payment. 4. Paid under OPPS; Separate APC payment.
L	Influenza vaccine; pneumococcal pneumonia vaccine	Not paid under OPPS. Paid at reasonable cost; Not subject to deductible or coinsurance.
M	Items and services not billable to the fiscal intermediary	Not paid under OPPS.
N	Items and services packaged into APC rates	Paid under OPPS; Payment is packaged into payment for other services, including outliers. Therefore, there is no separate APC payment.
P	Partial Hospitalization	Paid under OPPS; Per diem APC payment.

(Continued)

Table 2.1 Status indicators (*continued*)

Indicator	Item/Code/Service	OPPS Payment Status
Q	Packaged services subject to separate payment under OPPS payment criteria.	Paid under OPPS; Addendum B displays APC assignments when services are separately payable. 1. Separate APC payment based on OPPS payment criteria. 2. If criteria are not met, payment is packaged into payment for other services, including outliers. Therefore, there is no separate APC payment.
S	Significant procedure, not discounted when multiple	Paid under OPPS; Separate APC payment.
T	Significant procedure, multiple reduction applies	Paid under OPPS; Separate APC payment.
V	Clinic or emergency department visit	Paid under OPPS; Separate APC payment.
X	Ancillary services	Paid under OPPS; Separate APC payment.
Y	Nonimplantable durable medical equipment	Not paid under OPPS. All institutional providers other than home health agencies bill to DMERC.

Discounting Computation

When two or more significant surgical procedures are performed in one encounter, the payment for the second procedure may be discounted. Because the overall payment rate for a procedure includes all items normally performed by the primary procedure, it would be inaccurate to pay the full value for two procedures when they are performed together. For this reason, the OPPS system includes a provision for discounting. If two or more procedures performed have been assigned a status indicator of "T," they are subject to the discounting rule. This means that the first or most extensive procedure will be paid at the full value of the APC group rate, but the secondary T procedure will be discounted by 50 percent. All non-T procedures performed in the encounter and coded will be paid according to their status indicator and other payment rules.

Inpatient Only Procedures

When establishing the OPPS system, Medicare reviewed all procedures from a clinical nature to determine which should be paid under the payment methodology for outpatient procedures. Because many of the CPT procedures identify those that are more likely to be performed in the inpatient setting, a list was developed that includes those that would not be paid as an outpatient. These inpatient only procedures are indicated by Status Indicator "C." If these procedures are performed in the outpatient setting, Medicare will not reimburse the facility for any related services performed during that encounter. Each year this list is refined and if a procedure is deemed appropriate to be performed in the outpatient setting, the procedure code is removed from the inpatient only list and receives a new status indicator as appropriate.

Services already paid on a fee schedule or other predetermined rate will not be paid under OPPS. Some of these are screening mammograms, laboratory services, professional services of physicians, and ESRD services.

Weights and Payments

Similar to the IPPS system, all APC groups are assigned a weight based on the group's resource usage compared with the average usage for Medicare patients. Although inpatients are placed into one DRG category during their hospitalization, under OPPS, patients may receive several services that are payable under separate APC groups.

CCI Edits

Correct coding initiative (CCI) edits are included in the Medicare payment software known as the Outpatient Code Editor (OCE). These edits are used to identify claims that contain multiple procedure codes that may not need to be paid separately. There are two main types of edits. The most common of these is the comprehensive or component edits where one code is considered to be a component of another code. If both codes are used, only the more comprehensive code is paid.

Mutually exclusive edits cover code combinations when one of the codes is considered improbable or impossible to be performed with the other code. These edits also encompass codes that are billed together when one code includes "with" services and the other billed code is "without" the same certain services. The edits are set to pay the least expensive code.

Medical Visits

To assign APCs to medical visits, Medicare requires hospitals to use CPT Evaluation and Management (E/M) codes to identify clinic and emergency department visits. These codes were designed to capture physician professional billing and were not intended for use by hospitals for facility services. Hospitals were instructed to map their current methodology used to capture staffing in these departments to the CPT codes and to create a standardized procedure to uniformly assign the codes.

Hospitals may receive additional payment for other services performed with the medical visit, such as diagnostic testing, infusion of drugs, therapeutic procedures including respiration, and certain expensive medications such as "clot buster" drugs used for stroke and heart attack patients.

Annual Review of System

APC groups, weights, wage, and other adjustments are reviewed on an annual basis to account for changes in technology, HCPCS codes, medical practice, new services, cost data, and other considerations. An expert panel consisting of provider representatives is consulted during this annual review. The OPPS is maintained on a calendar year basis so that new payment rates coincide with revisions to the CPT and HCPCS Level II code updates effective on January 1 of each year.

Payment for Physicians: Resource-Based Relative Value System/Scale

In 1984, Medicare placed a fee hold on physician payment because of increasing costs. CMS began requiring the use of CPT codes in 1985 for payment on a fee schedule basis, and in 1989 they required the usage of ICD-9-CM codes for physician billing. In 1992, physicians began to be paid through a PPS known as Resource-Based Relative Value System/Scale or RBRVS. A fee schedule is published each year that displays the amount that physicians will be paid for their services. As ICD-10-CM is implemented, these code requirements will shift to reflect ICD-10-CM diagnosis codes needed to justify the procedures being performed and paid through CPT or HCPCS codes. Physicians will not use ICD-10-PCS for coding procedures, but will continue to use the CPT or HCPCS coding systems.

Procedures are coded utilizing the CPT or HCPCS coding systems. Under the RBRVS, each code is assigned three separate relative value units (RVUs), or weights, to account for resource use and complexity of service for the procedure. Those three areas are calculated based on work value, practice expense (PE), and malpractice cost (MP) and are adjusted for each geographic area. Calculations are set to include fees for each test and the value of services such as history taking, consultation with other doctors and explanation of findings. The three RVUs are adjusted for each region to account for variations in the cost of operating medical practices in different parts of the country. This is known as the geographic practice cost index (GPCI). It is important that the place of service be entered onto the physician billing form correctly, because payment may be different for various sites of care, such as hospital, physician clinic, or nursing home. For example, if a procedure is performed in the physician's clinic, that physician has overhead costs including costs of supplies. If the same procedure is performed in a hospital setting, the physician typically does not have to incur the cost of supplies, making the cost to the physician lower and reducing payment. The conversion factor (CF) is a base dollar amount that is set for that fiscal year. To determine the final amount that a physician will be paid for a service, the CF is multiplied by all three RVUs.

The formula for calculating 2013 physician fee schedule payment amount is displayed in figure 2.1.

Figure 2.1 Calculating 2013 physician fee schedule payment

2013 Non-Facility Pricing Amount = [(Work RVU * Work GPCI) + (Transitioned Non-Facility PE RVU * PE GPCI) + (MP RVU * MP GPCI)] * Conversion Factor (CF)

2013 Facility Pricing Amount = [(Work RVU * Work GPCI) + (Transitioned Facility PE RVU * PE GPCI) + (MP RVU * MP GPCI)] * CF

The Conversion Factor for CY 2013 is $34.0230

Notes:

RVU is the abbreviation for Relative Value Unit

GPCI = Geographic practice cost index

PE = Practice Expense

MP = Malpractice costs

Source: http://www.cms.hhs.gov/center/provider-type/physician-center.html

---

Other Insurance Programs

This section addresses other insurance programs like Medicaid, military programs, and group insurance plans.

Medicaid

Medicaid was established in 1965 by Public Law 89-97 (Title XIX of the Social Security Act) as a jointly funded program between the state and federal governments. The program was set up to care for low-income or indigent patients. Although it is federally funded, the program is run primarily by the individual states. Eligibility, services provided, and payment rates vary from state to state, but the programs must meet general national guidelines for services. The CMS Medicaid Eligibility Summary defines the following categories of patients as eligible for Medicaid:

- Individuals who meet the requirements for the Aid to Families with Dependent Children (AFDC) program that was in effect in their state on July 16, 1996
- Children younger than age six years whose family income is at or below 133 percent of the federal poverty level (FPL)
- Pregnant women whose family income is below 133 percent of the FPL (services to these women are limited to those related to pregnancy, complications of pregnancy, delivery, and postpartum care)
- Supplemental Security Income (SSI) recipients in most states (some states use more restrictive Medicaid eligibility requirements that predate SSI)
- Recipients of adoption or foster care assistance under Title IV of the Social Security Act
- Special protected groups (typically individuals who lose their cash assistance due to earnings from work or from increased Social Security benefits, but who may keep Medicaid for a period of time)
- All children who are younger than age 19 years, in families with incomes at or below the FPL
- Certain Medicare beneficiaries, such as those with low income

Some states have received permission from the federal government to make modifications to the basic Medicaid plans to include uninsurable individuals, the "medically needy," and children.

Military Programs

TRICARE (formerly known as the Civilian Health and Medical Program of the Uniformed Services [CHAMPUS]) provides medical coverage for active duty and retired service members. This coverage applies to members of the seven uniformed services (Army, Air Force, Navy, Marine Corps, Coast Guard, Public Health Service, and the National Oceanic and Atmospheric Administration) and their dependents, as well as individuals whose spouses were killed in action.

TRICARE pays for coverage in facilities other than military hospitals and offers several options, including an HMO type of coverage system and a fee-based payment system. The HMO/managed care option is known as TRICARE Prime. TRICARE Extra allows TRICARE beneficiaries to make appointments with civilian practitioners who participate by accepting the TRICARE maximum allowable amount as payment in full, and TRICARE Standard is a fee-for-service plan. TRICARE Plus is a variation of the plan used to cover services in military healthcare facilities when available.

For beneficiaries who are Medicare eligible (age 65 years and older), there is also a TRICARE for Life plan option. This plan works as a secondary insurance for those who have Medicare Part B. It picks up expenses, such as coinsurance and deductible costs, after Medicare pays its portion of the bill.

TRICARE for Life uses a DRG-modified system to reimburse facilities for inpatient care. This benefit is available only when the patient is in the hospital for more days than are allowable under the Medicare system. For days 151 and later of a Medicare stay, TRICARE reimburses the hospital the DRG amount minus the patient's additional copayment rate, which is approximately 25 percent of the charges if the hospital is in-network. It is important to keep in mind that as Medicare updates its DRG payment system, users of the data will make updates to their payment systems as well.

The healthcare plan for veterans is the Civilian Health and Medical Program of the Department of Veterans Affairs (CHAMPVA). This plan consists of comprehensive coverage where both the veteran and the Veterans Administration (VA) pay a portion of covered healthcare expenses.

According to the Department of Veterans Affairs, CHAMPVA is a healthcare benefits program for the spouse or widow(er) and for the children of a veteran who:

1. Is rated by a VA regional office as permanently and totally disabled due to a service connected disability.
2. Was rated as permanently and totally disabled due to a VA rated service connected condition at the time of death.

3. Died of a VA rated service connected disability.

4. Died in the line of duty, not due to misconduct and the dependents are not otherwise eligible for Department of Defense TRICARE benefits.

In addition, a Medicare secondary plan called CHAMPVA For Life is available for those covered beneficiaries who are age 65 years and older. These patients must have Medicare benefits because CHAMPVA is always a secondary payer to Medicare. See the VA website for more information.

Commercial and Nonprofit Group Medical Insurance Plans

Group medical insurance plans are usually purchased through or by an employer. Some patients who cannot qualify for individual insurance plans because of preexisting conditions can obtain insurance through employer-sponsored group plans.

Self-employed individuals or those who work in a group that does not provide group insurance may be eligible to obtain individual medical insurance. These types of policies may cost more than group plans and may contain strict regulations, such as a preexisting conditions clause. Patients who have medical conditions deemed to have existed at the time of coverage do not receive benefits related to those preexisting conditions for a specified time frame after coverage begins.

Insurance companies provide various types of healthcare coverage options and benefits for their customers. For example, a review of a major Blue Cross and Blue Shield program shows that it offers the following options:

- *Major medical:* This option is usually a fee-for-service plan as discussed earlier. Although patients enjoy greater flexibility in the types of services and the number of providers from which to choose, major medical plans tend to be the most expensive for the patient, with higher deductibles and out-of-pocket expenses.

- *Preferred payment plan:* The preferred payment plan is a PPO type system where members have a more limited number of providers to select from negotiated contracts with the facilities and physician practices. They may include a point of service (POS) option, allowing the beneficiary to go out of network for a reduced percentage of reimbursement.

- *Hospital reimbursement program:* The hospital reimbursement program is used for reimbursement for hospital inpatient stays. The hospital agrees to accept a DRG-type payment methodology where the payment received is considered as payment in full. The beneficiary will incur no costs other than the deductible and copayment amounts. This plan is similar to the DRG system utilized in the Medicare inpatient PPS.

- *COBRA benefits:* Patients who have group insurance and leave their jobs or are laid off are usually eligible to keep their insurance coverage up to 18 months after their employment ends, but are required to pay the premiums required to keep the coverage intact. These benefits are provided by federal law under the Consolidated Omnibus Budget Reconciliation Act (COBRA) of 1986. Continuation of coverage is only effective under specific circumstances, such as loss of a job or life events such as death or divorce. Typically, COBRA is in effect for employers who offer group healthcare and have 20 or more employees.

- *HIPAA benefits:* The Health Insurance Portability and Accountability Act (HIPAA) of 1996 allows for healthcare coverage protection for those who move or change jobs, although the premiums for these policies are often very expensive. HIPAA also prohibits group plans from either denying coverage or charging extra because of current or past medical history. There is usually a limited or no preexisting conditions clause in the HIPAA insurance plan. Patients have to show that they have a minimum of 18 months of credible coverage of previous insurance without significant break (no more than 63 consecutive days without insurance) to be eligible for HIPAA insurance.

Forms Overview: Billing Forms and Their Components and Fields Explained

The National Uniform Claim Committee (NUCC) and the National Uniform Bill Committee are made up of representatives from both providers and health insurance organizations and are responsible for maintaining and updating the standardized forms used in billing of healthcare claims. The form used to bill for physician professional services (Medicare Part B Claims) is known as the CMS-1500 form and the standardized form used in billing hospital (Medicare Part A) claims is called the Uniform Billing-04 (UB-04). These forms are standardized in order to be utilized for billing claims for all payers. While most claims are sent electronically, there are still some occasions where a paper claim can be utilized. Hospitals (facilities) submit electronic claims via the 8371 electronic format which has replaced the UB-04 paper billing form. Physicians (providers) submit claims via either the 837P electronic format or the CMS-1500 paper billing form. Data elements in the CMS uniform electronic billing specifications are consistent with the hard copy data set to the extent that one processing system can handle both.

CMS-1500

The CMS-1500 form (figure 2.2) is maintained by the NUCC and is the standardized claim form used for billing physician professional services when a paper claim is allowed. This form was updated primarily to accommodate the National Provider Identifier (NPI), an updated unique provider number that was required by the HIPAA law. The NUCC maintains a crosswalk between the electronic form and the 1500 paper format.

Hospital Billing Formats

The 8371 is the standard format utilized by hospitals and other institutional providers to electronically transmit healthcare claims. The UB-04 (figure 2.3), also known as the CMS-1450 form, is used for billing when paper claims are allowed. The UB-04 is maintained by the National Uniform Billing Committee (NUBC). According to the CMS website, "The NUBC is a voluntary, multidisciplinary committee that develops data elements for claims and claim-related transactions and it is composed of all major national provider and payer organizations (including Medicare). The American Hospital Association facilitates its meetings." See the CMS website for an explanation of the billing process for hospital inpatient services.

Figure 2.2 CMS-1500 form

Figure 2.3 Uniform Billing-04/CMS-1450 form

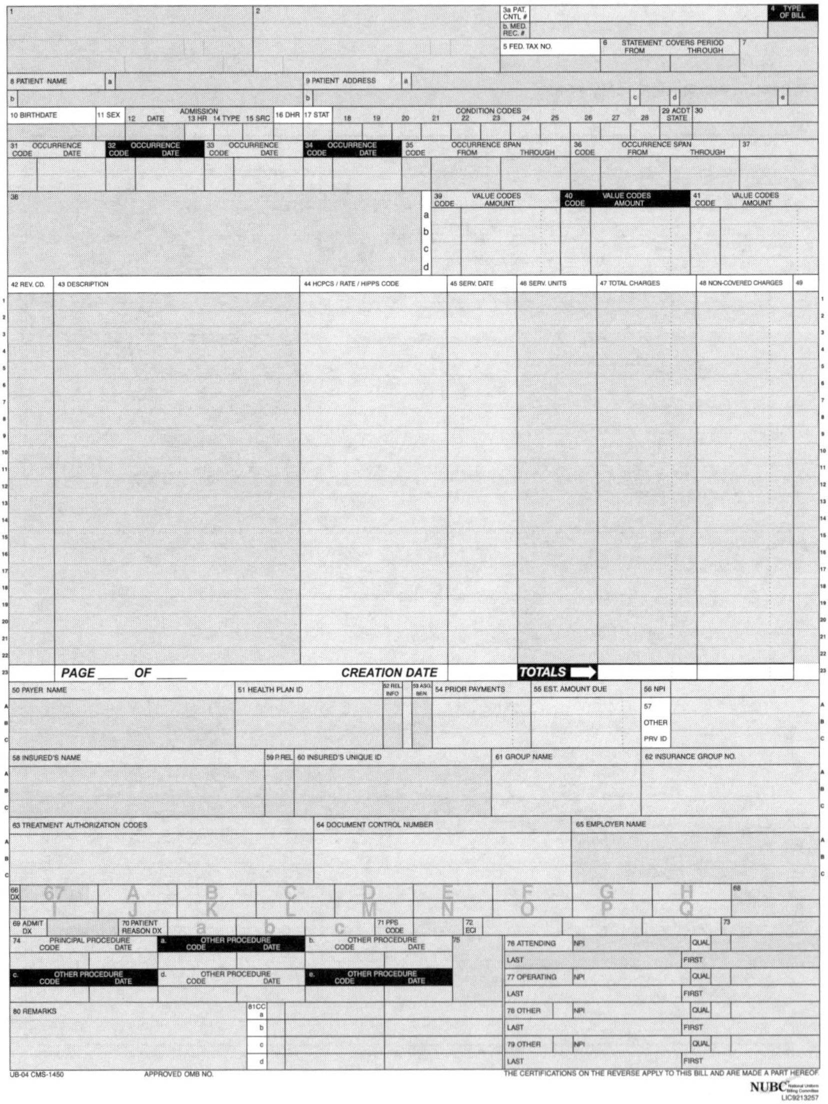

1 | 2 | 3a PAT. CNTL # | b. MED. REC. # | 4 TYPE OF BILL
5 FED. TAX NO. | 6 STATEMENT COVERS PERIOD FROM THROUGH | 7
8 PATIENT NAME a b | 9 PATIENT ADDRESS a b c d e
10 BIRTHDATE | 11 SEX | ADMISSION 12 DATE 13 HR 14 TYPE 15 SRC | 16 DHR | 17 STAT | CONDITION CODES 18 19 20 21 22 23 24 25 26 27 28 | 29 ACDT STATE | 30
31 OCCURRENCE CODE DATE | 32 OCCURRENCE CODE DATE | 33 OCCURRENCE CODE DATE | 34 OCCURRENCE CODE DATE | 35 OCCURRENCE SPAN CODE FROM THROUGH | 36 OCCURRENCE SPAN CODE FROM THROUGH | 37
38 | 39 VALUE CODES CODE AMOUNT | 40 VALUE CODES CODE AMOUNT | 41 VALUE CODES CODE AMOUNT | a b c d
42 REV. CD. | 43 DESCRIPTION | 44 HCPCS / RATE / HIPPS CODE | 45 SERV. DATE | 46 SERV. UNITS | 47 TOTAL CHARGES | 48 NON-COVERED CHARGES | 49
1–23
PAGE ____ OF ____ | CREATION DATE | TOTALS
50 PAYER NAME | 51 HEALTH PLAN ID | 52 REL. INFO | 53 ASG. BEN. | 54 PRIOR PAYMENTS | 55 EST. AMOUNT DUE | 56 NPI | 57 OTHER PRV ID | A B C
58 INSURED'S NAME | 59 P.REL | 60 INSURED'S UNIQUE ID | 61 GROUP NAME | 62 INSURANCE GROUP NO. | A B C
63 TREATMENT AUTHORIZATION CODES | 64 DOCUMENT CONTROL NUMBER | 65 EMPLOYER NAME | A B C
66 DX | 67 A B C D E F G H I J K L M N O P Q | 68
69 ADMIT DX | 70 PATIENT REASON DX a b c | 71 PPS CODE | 72 ECI | 73
74 PRINCIPAL PROCEDURE CODE DATE | a. OTHER PROCEDURE CODE DATE | b. OTHER PROCEDURE CODE DATE | 75
c. OTHER PROCEDURE CODE DATE | d. OTHER PROCEDURE CODE DATE | e. OTHER PROCEDURE CODE DATE
76 ATTENDING NPI QUAL LAST FIRST
77 OPERATING NPI QUAL LAST FIRST
80 REMARKS | 81CC a b c d
78 OTHER NPI QUAL LAST FIRST
79 OTHER NPI QUAL LAST FIRST
UB-04 CMS-1450 | APPROVED OMB NO. | THE CERTIFICATIONS ON THE REVERSE APPLY TO THIS BILL AND ARE MADE A PART HEREOF.
NUBC National Uniform Billing Committee LIC9213257

Chapter 3

Coding Compliance

Fraud and Abuse

The United States government has established a defined group, with oversight by the Office of the Inspector General (OIG) of the Department of Health and Human Services (HHS), to investigate areas of fraud and abuse in the healthcare industry. The OIG works with the United States Department of Justice, which includes the Federal Bureau of Investigation (FBI) and the United States Attorney's Offices, to investigate and prosecute violations of the law. These groups also work at the individual state level with private insurance carriers, states' attorneys general, state Medicaid fraud units, fiscal intermediaries, and Medicare Part B carriers to evaluate allegations of fraud and abuse.

According to the OIG, facilities should participate voluntarily in programs designed to maintain compliance with all billing and coding regulations. To assist with this process, the OIG has published compliance program guidance for several different types of healthcare entities, including hospitals. In conjunction with the Centers for Medicare and Medicaid Services (CMS), the FBI, and other federal and state agencies, the OIG works to detect fraud and abuse in the healthcare industry.

This chapter examines the programs and policies involved in ensuring coding compliance. It also describes the components of a facility compliance plan.

Fraud and abuse consist of the acts of providers that are deemed to have defrauded the government or abused the right to bill for services rendered. Fraudulent activity means that the provider intentionally, or with reckless disregard for the truth, filed false healthcare claims. These findings can result in civil or criminal prosecution. Erroneous claims, or abuse, are innocent billing errors that result in the minimum of return of overpayments or funds received in error.

Federal Civil False Claims Act

The Federal Civil False Claims Act (FCA) (31 USC§3729–3733) is the legislation that provides the framework for federal fraud and abuse penalties and investigations. It defines liability for anyone who knowingly files a fraudulent claim with the intention of obtaining inappropriate funds from the government. The law specifies that a claim of fraud can be made up to 10 years from the date of violation.

The phrase "knew or should have known" is frequently used in conjunction with fraud and abuse. Professionals and facilities are required to adhere to all published rules and guidance. Whether they actually knew about a certain rule does not matter; if the rule was published, it should be followed.

OIG Guidance for Compliance Programs

The OIG publishes studies and recommendations for program adjustments to prevent fraud and reduce waste and abuse. Additionally, it issues special fraud alerts to notify the public and healthcare community about schemes in the provision of healthcare services.

The OIG Work Plan

Each year, the OIG publishes a plan that outlines projects and issues that will be studied during the upcoming fiscal year. According to the OIG website,

> The OIG Work Plan sets forth various projects to be addressed during the fiscal year by the Office of Audit Services, Office of Evaluation and Inspections, Office of Investigations, and Office of Counsel to the Inspector General. The work plan includes projects planned in each of the Department's major entities: the Centers for Medicare & Medicaid Services; the public health agencies; and the Administrations for Children, Families, and Aging. Information is also provided on projects related to issues that cut across departmental programs, including State and local government use of Federal funds, as well as the functional areas of the Office of the Secretary. Some of the projects described in the Work Plan are statutorily required, such as the audit of the Department's financial statements, which is mandated by the Government Management Reform Act.

The OIG begins its work plan year by discussing projects on areas that have been identified as having potential for fraudulent activities. As the year progresses, studies and projects may be added to the plan as other problematic areas are identified. The work plan is divided into the specific guidance concerning hospitals, home health, nursing homes, and hospice. A separate section discusses areas of concern for physician professional billing, medical equipment companies, and other billing areas including Part B drug coverage and managed care. Because the OIG oversees all government payment systems, there are separate issues identified under Medicare, Medicaid, and public health agencies.

OIG reports focus on program audits and inspections, investigative focus areas, and legal counsel focus areas. Fraud alerts and special reports are made available so that healthcare entities can utilize this information in order to assess their own compliance practices. It is recommended that healthcare organizations study the OIG work plans as they are published and incorporate topics of concern into their compliance plan for that time period. Fraud alerts and reports of potential fraudulent areas of concern should be monitored and internal practices evaluated on a regular basis. To view the current OIG work plan, see the OIG website.

Compliance Plan Guidance

In the *Federal Register*, published on February 23, 1998, the government issued guidance for compliance programs for hospitals. The OIG stated, "the adoption and implementation of voluntary compliance programs significantly advance the prevention of fraud, abuse, and waste in these healthcare plans while at the same time furthering the fundamental mission of all hospitals, which is to provide quality care to all patients." Since that time, the OIG has established sample compliance plans for various types of healthcare facilities including physician professional services, ambulance and pharmaceuticals, nursing facilities, and third party billing companies. These voluntary compliance plans help facilities to ensure that they are working to foster a compliance-focused atmosphere where all employees, physicians, and administration staff are educated and held accountable for their actions. Although the OIG work plan should be incorporated into compliance training and evaluation for each year, the facility's compliance plan should be designed as a more permanent document.

Even though there are some differences between compliance plans in different types of healthcare facilities, the OIG has identified seven key elements that were established as guidelines for an effective compliance program. A facility should

- Establish written policies, procedures, and standards of conduct
- Designate a chief compliance officer and appropriate committee(s)
- Provide an effective training and education program
- Develop effective communication and a process for reporting compliance issues

- Enforce the program through well-publicized disciplinary guidelines
- Audit and monitor the program
- Respond promptly to allegations by taking corrective action

Other sample compliance plans can be found on the OIG website.

Recovery Audit Contractors (RACs)

One of the newest initiatives by the government to eliminate fraud and abuse and recoup incorrect payments is found in the usage of Recovery Audit Contractors (RACs). These contractors are auditing charts to identify Medicare over- and underpayments and return incorrect payments to the government. These RACs are paid based on a percentage of money they identify and collect on behalf of the government. RACs are working to identify incorrect past Medicare payments and helping to prevent future overpayments to providers.

RACs primarily review areas such as medical necessity, excessive or duplicate payments, and Medicare secondary payer issues. The RAC demonstration program was successful in returning dollars to the Medicare Trust Fund and identifying monies that need to be returned to providers. It provided the Centers for Medicare and Medicaid Services (CMS) with a new mechanism for detecting improper payments made in the past and has also given CMS a valuable new tool for preventing future inappropriate payments, and the program was expanded to all 50 states. Each RAC is responsible for identifying overpayments and underpayments in approximately a quarter of the country. The RAC jurisdictions match Medicare administrative contractors (DME MACs) jurisdictions.

The CMS website contains updated information on the RAC jurisdiction map, schedule, and contractor information.

Standards of Ethical Coding

The American Health Information Management Association (AHIMA) has developed a set of guidelines for correct coding in its Standards of Ethical Coding, found as Appendix A of this text. All healthcare organizations should adopt these standards as a part of their compliance program.

Policies and Procedures

Definitive policies and procedures should be established and maintained to ensure that all members of the organization are following the guidelines. Comprehensive policies and procedures should include accurate coding, documentation, retention, contracts, and outsourcing. Internal coding practices should be well written, clear, and indicative that the facility follows official coding guidelines. Written coding accuracy standards and commitment should be in place to provide adequate coding resources for all coding staff.

Moreover, the policies and procedures should be used to identify and target possible areas of risk. Some of the most common areas of risk include

- Unbundling or fragmenting a service by reporting separate codes for services that are included in one procedure code
- Downcoding a service in order to assign an additional code (this also can occur by inappropriately separating the surgical approach from the major surgical service performed)

Other areas of concern are as follows:

- Diagnosis or procedure misrepresentation
- Assignment of a code for a higher level of service than the service provided
- Medically unnecessary diagnostic tests
- Inappropriate billing for teaching physicians
- Discrepancies between the physician's and hospital's codes

The policies and procedures should be communicated on a regular basis. A code of conduct should be developed that indicates a firm commitment to compliance as part of the daily routine and course of business.

Components of a Compliance Plan

The basic components of a compliance plan include designation of a compliance officer, training and education, communication strategies, auditing and monitoring activities, corrective action, and follow-up measures. In addition, mechanisms to ensure accurate and complete documentation in the health record must be in place to ensure coding and billing compliance.

Designation of a Compliance Officer

With the Compliance Program Guidance (CPG), the government recognized that facilities may have different needs in developing their compliance plan. The government recommends that organizations appoint a chief compliance officer and establish a compliance committee to provide assistance and guidance, as needed.

Training and Education

Training and education is a key component of all compliance plans. There should be mandatory annual training for new hires, professional staff, and physicians. Regular meetings should be held with coding staff to ensure compliance with any new rules and regulations. Focused training sessions should take place as problematic areas are identified, and compliance should be included in all performance evaluations. Facilities should establish job descriptions and qualification requirements for coding professionals and billing staff.

Communication

Communication is an essential component in all compliance plans. A mechanism must be in place for reporting perceived compliance violations. If employees think that their complaints will be ignored or used against them in some way, they will not report problems. They need to know that compliance is not just a requirement from the government but a part of the culture of the facility. No member or group can be exempt from the system.

Auditing and Monitoring

Another key component of a thorough compliance program is auditing. Auditing of the entire revenue cycle from patient service to payment should be completed on a regular basis. Some basic auditing steps include the following:

- Use OIG target areas to ensure compliance with key efforts by the government to prevent fraud.
- Evaluate internal coding practices on a regular basis.
- Compare internal findings with external benchmarking practices.

Frequency, scope, and size depend on the organization. There is no one size fits all compliance plan. It should be developed and reviewed on an ongoing basis to ensure that it is working properly and appropriately.

Corrective Action and Follow-Up

With any compliance issues that are identified, corrective action and follow-up must occur in a timely manner. Although timely may vary depending on the scope of the problem, it is commonly recommended that corrective measures be taken within 60 days of the date the complaint is reported. If employees think that their concerns are ignored, they are less likely to report possible violations in the future.

As healthcare organizations work to maintain and promote compliance in their facilities, they should examine several areas. These include comparison of coding and billing patterns, monitoring and evaluation of denials, and implementation of coding updates.

Monitor and Understand the Case-Mix Index

One area of concern for hospitals is the case-mix index (CMI). The CMI is the average diagnosis-related group (DRG) weight for a set of patients for a given time period. A CMI close to 1.000 shows that the facility's patients are using approximately the same amount of resources as the average Medicare patient. A higher CMI indicates patients who are more acutely ill than the average Medicare patient. As the government monitors submitted data in the Medicare Provider Analysis and Review Med PAR database, a hospital with a CMI that is statistically higher than that of surrounding areas may raise concern. In the early days of fraud and abuse investigations, several hospitals with unusually high CMIs were found to have improper coding and billing practices. See table 3.1 for CMI examples based on population and facility size.

The CMI should be calculated and tracked over time to allow the facility to monitor unusual events that have an impact on the overall CMI. For example, one or two highly weighted DRGs (such as Medicare Severity-Adjusted Diagnosis-Related Group 002 [MS-DRG 002] with a relative weight

Table 3.1 CMI examples

Population	CMI
Large urban areas (population > 1 million)	1.02
Other urban areas (population < 1 million)	1.04
Rural hospitals	0.84
Bed Size (Urban Facilities)	**CMI**
0–99 beds	0.91
100–199 beds	0.93
200–299 beds	1.00
300–499 beds	1.08
500 or more beds	1.17

of 13.97) will create an abnormally high CMI. When this happens, a high CMI does not accurately reflect the amount of resources used by the average patient in the facility.

Compare Utilization and Billing Patterns

A common practice is to benchmark against other facilities with similar traits, such as bed size and patient mix, physician specialty or types of services provided. This practice allows the organization to evaluate its performance statistics in comparison with like organizations and review any unusual findings. The benchmarks can then be compared to national, state, and regional norms.

Compare Coding and Billing Patterns Over Time

Facilities can also benchmark internally. The facility might use a simple graph to chart patterns over different time periods to determine problematic areas. It also should look for areas of concern, such as an unusually high CMI or a drop in reimbursement.

Monitor Claims Denials and Error Reports

As much as possible, facilities should have staff dedicated to monitoring all denials and claims that are returned to the provider (RTP). A simple spreadsheet, as shown in table 3.2, can be developed to monitor denials to evaluate areas for education and improvement in coding and billing practices.

Monitor Coding and DRG Changes

Facilities should monitor claims carefully in the first few months after coding changes take effect. These changes affect coding, billing, and documentation practices and should be reviewed to ensure that correct and complete claims are submitted. Some insurance companies may not have uploaded coding changes into their computer systems and may erroneously deny claims that make use of new codes.

Table 3.2 Example of denial spreadsheet

Reason for Denial	No. of Patients	$ Amount
Medical necessity	15	$4,345
Noncovered services	3	$2,356
CCI edits	5	$6,742

Appeal Inappropriate Denials

As denials are being monitored, it is imperative that incorrect or inappropriate denials be appealed.

Documentation Requirements

As discussed in other chapters, documentation in the health record is key to ensuring coding and billing compliance. According to Medicare, documentation should be available to the coder at the time of coding and sufficient to support the claim. It should be timely, with dictation and transcription completed as soon as possible after discharge. An established mechanism must be in place for obtaining physician clarification when the documentation is incomplete, illegible, or ambiguous so that billing accurately reflects the services provided.

Healthcare Quality Improvement Organizations

To ensure that the federal government pays only for medically necessary, appropriate, and high-quality healthcare services, CMS contracts with medical review organizations called quality improvement organizations (QIOs). These organizations were formerly known as peer review organizations. QIOs work with hospitals, physician practices, and other healthcare organizations in their area to conduct studies designed to help improve quality of care for Medicare beneficiaries. The QIOs' contract with CMS is known as the Scope of Work, a document that specifies the goals and topics for review. More information on the current work of the QIOs can be found at the CMS website.

Medicare Quality Initiative

Over the past several years, several quality initiatives have been implemented to address issues of poor quality in healthcare. 501(b) of the Medicare Modernization Act requires that certain inpatient hospitals submit quality data to the secretary of the HHS on a set of quality indicators in order to receive a full payment update. See figure 3.1 for a list of top indicators. Hospitals that do not submit data in the form and manner specified will have their payment update reduced.

The Hospital Value-based Purchasing Program began in fiscal year 2013 and applies to payments for discharges occurring on or after October 1, 2012. Under this program, CMS will make value-based incentive payments to acute care hospitals, based on either how well the hospitals perform on certain quality measures or how much the hospitals' performance improves

Figure 3.1 Top quality measures for inpatient hospitals

1. Heart attack (acute myocardial infarction)
   - Aspirin at arrival
   - Aspirin prescribed at discharge
   - Angiotensin-converting enzyme inhibitor (ACE-I) or angiotensin receptor blocker (ARB) for left ventricular systolic dysfunction
   - Beta blocker at arrival
   - Beta blocker prescribed at discharge
   - Fibrinolytic (thrombolytic) agent received within 30 minutes of hospital arrival
   - Percutaneous coronary intervention (PCI) received within 120 minutes of hospital arrival
   - Adult smoking cessation advice/counseling

2. Heart failure (HF)
   - Left ventricular function assessment
   - ACE-I or ARB for left ventricular systolic dysfunction
   - Discharge instructions
   - Adult smoking cessation advice/counseling

3. Pneumonia (PNE)
   - Initial antibiotic received within 4 hours of hospital arrival
   - Oxygenation assessment
   - Pneumococcal vaccination status
   - Blood culture performed before first antibiotic received in hospital
   - Adult smoking cessation advice/counseling
   - Appropriate initial antibiotic selection
   - Influenza vaccination status

4. Surgical Care Improvement Project (SCIP)
   - Prophylactic antibiotic received within 1 hour prior to surgical incision
   - Prophylactic antibiotic discontinued within 24 hours after surgery end time
   - SCIP-VTE 1: Venous thromboembolism (VTE) prophylaxis ordered for surgery patients
   - SCIP-VTE 2: VTE prophylaxis within 24 hours pre/post surgery
   - SCIP Infection 2: Prophylactic antibiotic selection for surgical patients

(Continued)

5. Mortality measures (Medicare patients)
- Acute Myocardial Infarction 30-day mortality (Medicare patients)
- Heart Failure 30-day mortality (Medicare patients)

6. Patients' experience of care
- HCAHPS patient survey

on certain quality measures from their performance during a baseline period. The higher a hospital's performance or improvement during the performance period for a fiscal year, the higher the hospital's value-based incentive payment for the fiscal year would be.

Hospitals are measured based on performance in two areas impacting quality: clinical process of care and patient experience of care. A total score for performance is assigned based on a weighting of these two factors.

More information on current government initiatives can be found on the CMS website.

Medicare is developing similar quality measures for outpatient, physician professional services, and other healthcare settings. It is important that professionals in all settings continue to evaluate their quality of care as one aspect of their compliance programs.

Chapter

4

Other Issues Impacting Coding

The Coding Process

Every healthcare facility should establish coding policies and procedures that establish guidelines for coding professionals to follow, ensuring coding consistency. Using the official coding guidelines established by the cooperating parties, guidelines and guidance provided by the American Hospital Association (AHA) and American Medical Association (AMA), and incorporating guidelines for facility-specific issues, well-developed policies can be instituted to increase coding accuracy and consistency.

The AHA publishes the official guidance for ICD-10-CM and ICD-10-PCS coding in a quarterly newsletter titled *Coding Clinic for ICD-10-CM and ICD-10-PCS* and *Coding Clinic for HCPCS* for assistance with HCPCS procedural coding. Prior to implementation of ICD-10, Coding Clinic for ICD-9-CM was published and should be reviewed for guidance on issues related to ICD-9-CM coding. Because this guidance is approved by the cooperating parties, these publications should be viewed as official sources for clarifying coding discrepancies. The AMA publishes information regarding CPT codes in a newsletter titled *CPT Assistant*. All of these publications can be used as a basis for developing facility policies and procedures.

Steps in the Coding Process

For accurate coding to occur, the coder must have a complete health record with clear documentation regarding the patient's encounter. Each facility needs to define what constitutes a complete record and whether that record is of an inpatient admission, outpatient encounter, or physician office visit. The coder must review the contents of the record to determine the patient's condition and the treatment and care received. Documentation in the entire patient health record should be reviewed to determine diagnoses and procedures that are appropriate for coding purposes. The coding process is similar to the job of an investigative reporter searching for the clues and details needed to tell the entire story. Coding is also like putting together a puzzle, searching for all the pieces to build a complete and accurate picture of the patient's diagnoses and treatments performed during the admission or encounter. It is important to note that the coder can only code what is clearly documented in the body of the patient health record. The coding process must be a joint effort between the professionals who document in the record and the coding professionals who must translate the documentation into medical codes. Because there are going to be times when the documentation is unclear, ambiguous, or incomplete, it is imperative that the facility establish a clear process for querying the physician(s) responsible for the documentation. (See the "Querying the Physician" section in this chapter.)

Inpatient Coding Process

Typically, the coding professional will begin the record review by reading the summary documentation. For an inpatient encounter, this usually begins with the discharge summary, which is written and dictated by the attending physician at the end of the patient's stay. This document summarizes the reasons for the patient's visit, the testing and procedure results, and the patient's response to treatment as well as the patient's disposition and future plan of care. By reviewing the discharge summary, the coder should gain an overall understanding of the main diagnoses and procedures performed during the hospital stay.

The other summary documentation, including the patient history and physical examination, and any operative reports, consultation reports, and progress notes help to fill in the details about the stay. The coder also reviews ancillary documentation such as laboratory, pathology, radiology, and cardiology results to determine other findings. These clues are used to validate the story that is told in the summary documents and also serve as the clinical information needed to help verify additional diagnoses or procedures. In the inpatient setting, the coder primarily uses the physician documentation to validate the code assignment. If other diagnoses or procedures are alluded to in the rest of the patient record, the coder may need to query the physician to determine if these findings hold enough clinical significance to justify coding. For example, if the coder notes that the patient had repeated laboratory values of low hematocrit and hemoglobin and was given four units of blood, the coding professional will query the physician to determine if the patient had an additional diagnosis of anemia, possibly linked to an acute blood loss, such as with gastrointestinal bleeding.

Outpatient Coding Process

An outpatient encounter includes any outpatient setting, including outpatient and emergency department episodes as well as physician office or clinic settings. For an outpatient encounter, the coder must review all documentation provided as part of that visit. A primary diagnosis, which is defined as the main reason for the visit, should be coded as well as any secondary diagnoses that impact the patient's care. In the outpatient setting, the coder is allowed to code from all documentation present during the coding process. If a test result is available, such as a pathology report or radiology report that is performed and authenticated by a physician, and a more definitive diagnosis is provided, then the coder is allowed to select the diagnosis for coding purposes. For example, if the ordering physician states that the patient is suffering from chest congestion and fever and the radiology report verifies that the patient has pneumonia, then the coding professional should select the diagnosis of pneumonia for coding purposes if the radiology report is available to the coder at the time of coding. However, if the patient's health record includes laboratory results showing hyperkalemia (a high potassium level), the coding professional must query the attending physician to determine if that test result is clinically significant. Laboratory tests are often performed by a computer or laboratory technician, and results may not be verified by a physician. In the outpatient setting, official coding guidelines state that "rule out," "suspected," or "probable" conditions cannot be coded. If only signs or symptoms are known definitively at the time of coding, then only those that are well documented are coded.

Preprinted forms such as fee or charge tickets, superbills, or encounter forms are used frequently in the outpatient setting (see figure 4.1). These forms include the most common diagnosis and procedure codes that describe provided services. Although these forms are helpful time-saving tools, they should be used with caution. Because a limited number of codes are available on the form, codes that provide details and specificity are not always included. Physicians or other healthcare personnel using these forms may only search for the term closest to describing the diagnosis or procedure that was performed, possibly leading to incorrect or generic coding. Because many insurance companies have limited numbers of diagnoses used to justify certain medical procedures, payment denials or payment delays may result. Typically, the preprinted form is considered to be a financial document and not part of the patient's legal health record. Documentation in the record must corroborate with the diagnoses or procedures marked on the form for billing of these services.

Figure 4.1 Example of preprinted form: Clinic charge ticket

INTERNAL MEDICINE SERVICES			D.O.S. _____
☐ CASH ☐ CHECK #	☐ CO-PAY	☐ RECEIPT #	AMT

Control #   SIGNED IN _____   APPT TIME _____

☐ WALK-IN   ☐ CONSULT   ☐ APPOINTMENT   TIME IN _____

PATIENT NAME (Last, First, MI)	SEX	SSN	DOB	Physician 1
				Physician 2
				Physician 3
ADDRESS	CITY	STATE	ZIP	Physician 4

PRIMARY INS: ☐ MEDICARE ☐ EDS ☐ COMM ☐ SELF-PAY ☐ PCP:
SECONDARY INS: ☐ MEDICARE ☐ EDS ☐ COMM ☐ SELF-PAY ☐ PCP:
ELIGIBLITY: APPROVED BY:

DX 1: _____   DX 2: _____   DX 3: _____   DX 4: _____

HEALTH CHECK SERVICES

DESCRIPTION	NEW PATIENT	ESTAB PATIENT	DX
☐ Infant 0-11 Months	☐ 99381	☐ 99391	V20.2
☐ 1 - 4 Years	☐ 99382	☐ 99392	V20.2
☐ 5 - 11 Years	☐ 99383	☐ 99393	V20.2
☐ 12 -17 Years	☐ 99384	☐ 99394	V20.2
☐ 18 - 39 Years	☐ 99385	☐ 99395	V70.0
☐ 40 - 64 Years	☐ 99386	☐ 99396	V70.0
☐ 65 Years and Older	☐ 99387	☐ 99397	V70.0

NEW PATIENTS		CODE	DX
☐ Level I - PF, PF, SF	10 min	☐ 99201	
☐ Level II - EPF, EPF, SF	20 min	☐ 99202	
☐ Level III - DET, DET, LOW	30 min	☐ 99203	
☐ Level IV - C, C, MOD	45 min	☐ 99204	
☐ Level V - C, C, HIGH	60 min	☐ 99205	

ESTABLISHED PATIENTS			DX
☐ Level I - MD not required	5 min	☐ 99211	
☐ Level II - PF, PF, SF	10 min	☐ 99212	
☐ Level III - EPF, EPF, LOW	15 min	☐ 99213	
☐ Level IV - DET, DET, MOD	25 min	☐ 99214	
☐ Level V - C, C, HIGH	40 min	☐ 99215	

OFFICE CONSULTATIONS			DX
☐ Level I - PF, PF, SF	15 min	☐ 99241	
☐ Level II - EPF, EPF, SF	30 min	☐ 99242	
☐ Level III - DET, DET, LOW	40 min	☐ 99243	
☐ Level IV - C, C, MOD	60 min	☐ 99244	
☐ Level V - C, C, HIGH	80 min	☐ 99245	

PROCEDURES		CODE	DX
Aspirate ganglion cyst		☐ 20612	
Aspirate/inject sm jt (fingers/toes)		☐ 20600	
Aspirate/inject intermed jt (wrist/elbow)		☐ 20605	
Aspirate/inject major joint (hip/knee)		☐ 20610	
Cerumen removal		☐ 69210	
Change burn dressing		☐ 16020	
Chemical cautery		☐ 17250	
I & D Abscess		☐ 10060	
I & D Hematoma		☐ 10140	
I & D Post Op Infection		☐ 10180	
Inject Tendon Sheath/Ligament		☐ 20550	
Inject Tendon Origin/Insertion		☐ 20551	
Inject Trigger Points (1-2)		☐ 20552	
Inject Trigger Points (3 or more)		☐ 20553	
Removal of Foreign Body	Ear	☐ 69200	
	Nose	☐ 30300	
	Eye	☐ 65205	
	Skin	☐ 10120	
Removal of Skin Tags (up to 15)		☐ 11200	
Removal of Skin Tags (additional 10)		☐ 11201+	
Wart Removal (1st wart)		☐ 17000	
Wart Removal (2-14 additional)		☐ 17003+	

INJECTIONS/MEDICATIONS	CODE	DX
Albuterol per 1 mg	☐ J7611	
Allergy Injection Single	☐ 95115	V07.1
Allergy Injection 2 or >	☐ 95117	V07.1
B-12 1000 mcg	☐ J3420	
Bicillin 1.2 mil units	☐ J0540	
Bicillin 2.4 mil units	☐ J0550	
D5W 1000cc	☐ J7070	
Depo Provera 150 mg	☐ J1055	V25.49
Imitrex	☐ J3030	
Insulin 5 units	☐ J1815	
Kenalog 10 mg	☐ J3301	
Rocephin 250 mg	☐ J0696	
Toradol 15 mg	☐ J1885	
Vancomycin 500 mg	☐ J3370	
Zithromax	☐ J0456	
Injection, SubQ/IM	☐ 90772	
IV, drip - 1st hr	☐ 90765	
IV, drip each additional hr	☐ 90766	
IV, push	☐ 90774	

LABORATORY	CODE	DX
Hemoglobin	☐ 85018	
Hematocrit	☐ 85014	
Occult Blood	☐ 82270	
One Touch Blood Glucose	☐ 82962	
Pap smear collection	☐ Q0091	V74.1
PPD Test	☐ 86580	
Pregnancy Test, Urine	☐ 81025	
Pulse Oximetry	☐ 94760	
Rapid Strep Test	☐ 87880	V74.1
Urinalysis	☐ 81002	
Wet Mount	☐ Q0111	
Wet Prep	☐ 87210	
Lab Handling	☐ 99000	
Venipuncture	☐ 36415	

EKG	CODE	DX
EKG, 12 lead total	☐ 93000	
EKG, tracing	☐ 93005	
EKG, intrepetation	☐ 93010	

AFTER HOURS/SPECIAL CARE	CODE	DX
After posted hours	☐ 99050+	
Other than office - special	☐ 99056+	
Emergency care in office	☐ 99058+	

IMMUNIZATIONS	CODE	DX
Hepatitis A	☐ 90632	V05.3
Hepatitis B Adult	☐ 90746	V05.3
Medicare Administration	☐ G0010	V05.3
Influenza Vaccine	☐ 90658	V04.81
Medicare Administration	☐ G0008	V04.81
MMR	☐ 90707	V06.4
Pneumovax Vaccine	☐ 90732	V03.82
Medicare Administration	☐ G0009	V03.82
Rubella	☐ 90706	V04.3
Td Adult	☐ 90718	V06.5
Tetanus Toxoid	☐ 90703	V03.7
Varicella	☐ 90716	V05.4
Vac Admin < 8 yrs of age with counseling, 1st	☐ 90465	
Vac Admin < 8 yrs of age with counseling, each additional	☐ 90466	
Vac Administration 1st	☐ 90471	
Vac Administration each additional vaccine	☐ 90472+	

PROCEDURES	CODE	DX
Lumbar puncture	☐ 62270	
MDI Teaching	☐ 94664	
Nebulizer Treatment	☐ 94640	
Pack anterior nasal hem.	☐ 30901	
Pack posterior nasal hem.	☐ 30905	
Simple Repair face, ears Less than 2.5 cm	☐ 12011	
2.6 cm to 5.0 cm	☐ 12013	
Simple Repair trunk, extremities Less than 2.5 cm	☐ 12001	
2.6 cm to 7.5 cm	☐ 12002	
Strapping, ankle	☐ 29540	
Strapping, elbow or wrist	☐ 29260	
Strapping, hand	☐ 29280	
Strapping, knee	☐ 29530	
Surgical Tray	☐ A4550	

WRITE IN SERVICES HERE: DX

Linking Diagnosis to Procedure

It is very helpful if the documentation clearly links all treatments to the diagnosis, condition, sign, or symptom that necessitated the treatment, especially in patients with multiple diagnoses or conditions identified during the episode of care. The Balanced Budget Act of 1997 requires physicians to provide a diagnosis to substantiate the necessity of any test that is performed by another entity (which can include a hospital, lab, or another physician). The diagnosis or other medical information should include the reason for the test, which can be a sign, symptom, or diagnosis.

A simple problem list of conditions can be created, such as,

- The patient had dysuria, so a urinalysis was ordered.
- The patient complained of chest pain, so an electrocardiogram was performed, which was normal.

Secondary Diagnosis Coding

Secondary diagnoses that impact the patient's care should be coded. For example, if a patient is treated for a urinary tract infection and is pregnant, both the pregnancy and the urinary tract infection should be coded. If a patient has a systemic or chronic disease that has the potential of complicating the patient's care, such as diabetes or chronic obstructive pulmonary disease, those secondary conditions should also be coded to build a more accurate picture of the patient's condition. Specific rules for assigning secondary codes are available in the official coding guidelines.

Querying the Physician

There are times when the coder needs to discuss the case with the attending physician because of unclear, ambiguous, or conflicting information in the patient's chart. According to the American Health Information Management Association (AHIMA) practice brief, "Managing an Effective Query Process" (found in Appendix B), the goal of the query process should be to improve physician documentation and coders' understanding of the unique clinical situation, not to improve reimbursement. Each facility should establish a policy and procedure for obtaining physician clarification of documentation that affects code assignment. The process of querying physicians must be a patient-specific process, not a general process. The practice brief "Guidelines for achieving a compliant query process" provides excellent examples of sample queries. It also reminds coders of appropriate reasons for querying the physician:

The generation of a query should be considered when the health record documentation

- Is conflicting, imprecise, incomplete, illegible, ambiguous, or inconsistent
- Describes or is associated with clinical indicators without a definitive relationship to an underlying diagnosis

- Includes clinical indicators, diagnostic evaluation, or treatment not related to a specific condition or procedure
- Provides a diagnosis without underlying clinical validation
- Is unclear for present on admission indicator assignment

Also according to the AHIMA practice brief, individuals who perform the query function should be familiar with the AHIMA standards of ethical coding (found in Appendix A), which direct coders to "assign and report only the codes and data that are clearly and consistently supported by health record documentation in accordance with applicable code set and abstraction conventions, rules, and guidelines." The standards further state:

> Query provider (physician or other qualified healthcare practitioner) for clarification and additional documentation prior to code assignment when there is conflicting, incomplete, or ambiguous information in the health record regarding a significant reportable condition or procedure or other reportable data element dependent on health record documentation (for example, present on admission indicator). (AHIMA 2013)

After the record is reviewed, the coder selects the diagnoses and procedures that need to be coded and assigns appropriate code numbers. Codes then have to be sequenced following appropriate guidelines including the definition of principal diagnosis for inpatient care (see Chapter 1 for more information). If a physician query is initiated, then the coding process is stopped until the physician has completed the documentation process. Typically, the coded data are entered into the clinical information system along with other data as part of an abstracting process. The coder or other trained healthcare professional carefully reviews the patient's documentation for other information required for reporting purposes, such as discharge disposition (where did the patient go when he or she left this facility) or quality indicators as required by Medicare, State Health reporting, or Healthcare Effectiveness Data and Information Set (HEDIS) reporting for physician practices.

These data then become the foundation for statistical, reimbursement, and clinical information systems. From a reimbursement standpoint, once all abstracted data are entered into the system, the data are placed onto the billing form in the correct data field to justify payment for the services provided. At this point, most facilities have a software program known as a "scrubber" that checks the claim for errors or potential discrepancies. If the software finds any issues, the claim is reviewed prior to sending to the insurance company. Once the discrepancies have been resolved, the claim is referred to as a clean claim. The billing form is then sent electronically or via mail to the insurance company or other third-party payer who then makes the determination to pay for those services. If there are any discrepancies or questions related to the information received, the payer may ask for more details about the items in question or may ask for copies of chart documentation to help decide the correct payment rate. Once all questions have been answered, payment is made for the services provided. The facility receives a statement from the payer that indicates the amount paid and reasons for any discounts or nonpayment of services. This statement is known as an Explanation of Benefits (EOB) or Remittance Advice (RA) in the hospital setting.

Quality Assessment for the Coding Process

Assessment of the coding process should occur through regular monitoring of coding accuracy. Monitoring is an ongoing internal review of coding practices conducted by an organization on a regular basis. A monitoring (or audit) program plan should include a written plan that outlines the objectives and frequency of the audits, record selection process, qualifications of auditors, and corrective actions the organization will take as a result of the audit findings.

Initially, a baseline audit should be performed. The audit should be a review of a large sample of the coding completed. It should include a sample of records coded by all coding professionals for all types of services. Moreover, the sample should be a representative of all physicians and types of cases treated by the organization. The baseline audit provides an overview of the organization's current coding practices.

The organization should conduct follow-up audits according to the schedule established in the monitoring or audit plan. Follow-up audits will provide ongoing monitoring of the coding process to ensure coding accuracy. The results of the audits also can be used to outline areas in which coding professional education and training are needed.

Clinical Documentation Improvement Program

Over the years, many facilities have struggled over when to begin the coding process. Traditionally, the chart is coded after the patient's encounter or episode of care is complete. If documentation is clear and complete, then the coder should have all the information needed to accurately assign codes to the patient's diagnoses and procedures. However, if the information is missing or ambiguous, obtaining answers to coding queries is difficult and time consuming once the patient has been discharged and the clinician has moved on to treating other patients. As Medicare and other payers look to improve the patient's care and provide more accurate payment based on the patient's documented severity of illness, organizations are retooling their coding process.

One such process is commonly known as a Clinical Documentation Improvement Program (CDIP). Coders work together with nursing staff or case managers to help ensure that clinical documentation is sufficient to support the patient's medical care. This process is designed to enhance patient care through better documentation. It also allows for a smoother coding process because any documentation issues are identified in "real time" instead of days or weeks after the patient has been treated.

Clinical documentation specialists (CDSs) are coding professionals and nurses who work on the patient floors or alongside the physicians in the clinic setting. Although some facilities may choose nursing staff for this position, coding professionals also are excellent candidates. It is imperative that the CDS has a mixture of coding and clinical knowledge and possesses the communication skills necessary to query physicians and other clinicians when questions arise regarding the medical documentation. In the physician clinic setting, the CDS may also review inpatient chart documentation to facilitate correct coding for the physician's professional services. This task also requires a strong working relationship between the hospital and physician practice. The CDI process will be especially important as facilities transition to ICD-10-CM and ICD-10-PCS as these systems are much more specific and may require additional documentation to fully identify the patient's conditions and procedures performed.

Other Uses of Coded Data

Although there is much discussion in this text regarding the use of coded data for reimbursement purposes, it is important to point out that this data is used for a variety of purposes. Historically, the data has been used as the basis for disease and procedure indices that provide facilities with a usable, searchable database to identify patterns of care, select cases for quality assurance activities, plan for service expansion, and conduct research. As mentioned in Chapter 2, quality indicators have been developed based on diagnosis codes to identify possible quality concerns. Some current uses of coded data were identified by AHIMA's Clinical Terminology and Classification Practice Council and are detailed in figure 4.2. Although this document refers to ICD-9-CM codes, they will be transitioned to the appropriate ICD-10-CM codes in the future.

Figure 4.2 Uses of coded data

Quality of Care Assessment

In 2001, the Agency for Healthcare Research and Quality (AHRQ) developed quality indicators that rely on hospital administrative data, including ICD-CM diagnosis codes, to construct a picture of the quality of medical care provided by a hospital and identify potential quality problems or success stories to be further investigated. Many state and regional hospital associations generate comparative data reports of these quality indicators as part of their quality programs and performance measurement systems.

An example of an AHRQ Inpatient Quality Indicator (IQI) is IQI 20, pneumonia mortality rate. This indicator monitors the number of deaths occurring for patients with a principal diagnosis of pneumonia. AHRQ selected the indicator because appropriate treatment with antibiotics is shown to result in reduced mortality rates from pneumonia.

Through the Joint Commissions' ORYX initiative facilities report coded data used to assess the quality of care provided to patients and to compare performance on these core measures to other facilities.

Patient Safety Evaluation

AHRQ developed Patient Safety Indicators (PSIs) as a screening tool to identify areas in which system or process changes could reduce preventable errors. Examples of PSI data tracked through coded data include obstetrical trauma in vaginal deliveries requiring instrumentation and cases of reclosure of postoperative disruption of abdominal surgical wounds. Currently, PSI data are used by various state agencies for safety monitoring and confidential internal analyses.

Risk Adjustment

In order to provide a fair evaluation of outcome data, many researchers are developing risk-adjustment methodologies. Many of the risk adjustment systems use ICD-9-CM data to classify patients into clinically meaningful groups and to further divide patients into severity-of-illness and risk-of-mortality subclasses. These risk adjustment tools are used to support a variety of data analysis efforts being conducted by individual healthcare facilities, state agencies, and hospital associations.

Pay-for-Performance Initiatives

Along with other care measures gathered through data abstraction, coded information is also being used for pay-for-performance initiatives. For example, in 2003, the Anthem Blue Cross and Blue

(Continued)

Shield of Virginia Quality Insights Hospital Incentive Program began aligning financial incentives with achievement on specific objectives. As part of the program, hospitals are required to select two of a subset of nine AHRQ PSIs for monitoring and root cause analysis, when appropriate. The Centers for Medicare & Medicaid Services (CMS) is also currently piloting pay-for-performance initiatives with hospitals and physicians. These programs link bonus payments on a variety of measures. For hospitals, this includes two of the PSIs.

Public Health Surveillance

Coded data play a critical role in identifying and tracking disease outbreaks and in routine epidemiological monitoring. Recently, the use of coded data for surveillance purposes is being explored more closely by public health specialists to detect and respond more effectively to bioterrorism threats.

Clinical Decision Support

Healthcare data are being used to activate clinical alerts, prevention and chronic disease reminders, and in clinical decision support. This expanded application of healthcare data in the care provision has further increased the importance of the accuracy and timeliness of these data.

Coded and abstracted data from health record documentation also serves as the foundation for many clinical decision support algorithms. For example, a decision support tool developed to identify patients at high risk for developing deep vein thrombosis (and thus in need of prophylaxis) searches data for ICD-9-CM codes indicating a history of venous thrombosis or embolism, recent trauma or surgery, or current conditions such as venous insufficiency or obesity. ICD-9-CM coded data are also being used to develop patient profiles for proprietary clinical decision support systems to check if any of the patient's current medical conditions could have been caused by a drug included on the patient's current medication list.

Source: AHIMA Clinical Terminology and Classification Practice Council, 2006.

Coding Professionals

Many coding professionals gain much of their coding knowledge on the job. It is imperative that the coder have a strong background in medical terminology and anatomy and physiology. At times, the coding system terminology may not match exactly with the physician terminology used to describe a procedure. The coder must act as a translator to interpret the chart documentation into an accurate code assignment. Because coding plays such a vital role in correct reimbursement, credentialed coders are in high demand. Although there are several organizations that provide credentialing opportunities for coders, AHIMA, as one of the cooperating parties, is seen as one of the top organizations that provides education and certification opportunities. AHIMA offers five certification examinations that test coding accuracy.

Health information management (HIM) professionals who have completed college or university degree programs accredited by the Commission on Accreditation for Health Informatics and Information Management Education (CAHIIM) take national examinations upon completion of their degrees.

Individuals with associate's degrees take a national examination to become Registered Health Information Technicians (RHITs). According to AHIMA's certification website,

> Professionals holding the RHIT credential are health information technicians who
>
> - Ensure the quality of medical records by verifying their completeness, accuracy, and proper entry into computer systems.
> - Use computer applications to assemble and analyze patient data for the purpose of improving patient care or controlling costs.
> - Often specialize in coding diagnoses and procedures in patient records for reimbursement and research. An additional role for RHITs is cancer registrars—compiling and maintaining data on cancer patients.
>
> With experience, the RHIT credential holds solid potential for advancement to management positions, especially when combined with a bachelor's degree.
>
> Although most RHITs work in hospitals, they are also found in other healthcare settings including office-based physician practices, nursing homes, home health agencies, mental health facilities, and public health agencies. In fact, RHITs may be employed in any organization that uses patient data or health information, such as pharmaceutical companies, law and insurance firms, and health product vendors. (AHIMA 2013)

HIM professionals who complete bachelor degree programs take an examination to become Registered Health Information Administrators (RHIAs). According to the AHIMA certification website,

Working as a critical link between care providers, payers, and patients, the RHIA

- Is an expert in managing patient health information and medical records, administering computer information systems, collecting and analyzing patient data, and using classification systems and medical terminologies.
- Possesses comprehensive knowledge of medical, administrative, ethical and legal requirements and standards related to healthcare delivery and the privacy of protected patient information.
- Manages people and operational units, participates in administrative committees, and prepares budgets.
- Interacts with all levels of an organization—clinical, financial, administrative, and information systems—that employ patient data in decision making and everyday operations.

Job opportunities for RHIAs exist in multiple settings throughout the healthcare industry. These include the continuum of care delivery organizations, including hospitals, multispecialty clinics and physician practices, long-term care, mental health, and other ambulatory care settings. The profession has seen significant expansion in nonpatient care settings, with careers in managed care and insurance companies, software vendors, consulting services, government agencies, education, and pharmaceutical companies. (AHIMA 2013)

Although the RHIT and RHIA examinations cover many areas relevant to their broad-based training, part of the examination tests clinical and coding knowledge skills. Because these examinations are designed to be taken after completing educational requirements, they test at an entry level of knowledge.

AHIMA also developed three examinations for coding professionals. The Certified Coding Associate (CCA) examination is considered to be an entry level examination, and according to the AHIMA certification website,

New coders who earn the CCA will immediately demonstrate their competency in the field, even if they don't have much job experience. Earning a CCA demonstrates a commitment to coding even for those who are new in the field. The CCA should be viewed as the starting point for an individual entering a new career as a coder.

The CCS or the Certified Coding Specialist-Physician Based (CCS-P) examinations demonstrate the mastery level skills that the CCA would strive for to advance his or her career:

Certified Coding Specialists (CCS) are professionals skilled in classifying medical data from patient records, generally in the hospital setting. These coding practitioners review patients' records and assign numeric codes for each diagnosis and procedure. To perform this task, they must possess expertise in the diagnosis coding system and the surgery section within the CPT coding system. In addition, the CCS is knowledgeable of medical terminology, disease processes, and pharmacology. The CCS credential demonstrates tested data quality and integrity skills in a coding practitioner. The CCS certification examination assesses mastery or proficiency in coding rather than entry-level skills.

The Certified Coding Specialist-Physician Based (CCS-P) is a coding practitioner with expertise in physician-based settings such as physician offices, group practices, multispecialty clinics, or specialty centers. This coding practitioner reviews patients' records and assigns numeric codes for each diagnosis and procedure. To perform this task, the individual must possess in-depth knowledge of the CPT coding system and familiarity with the current ICD diagnosis system and HCPCS Level II coding systems. The CCS-P is also expert in health information documentation, data integrity, and quality. Because patients' coded data is submitted to insurance companies or the government for expense reimbursement, the CCS-P plays a critical role in the health provider's business operation. (AHIMA 2013)

Shortage of Coding Professionals

Over the years, the market has continued to show a great need for coding professionals with a wealth of knowledge regarding coding and reimbursement. As these professionals take on new roles and more responsibility, it is evident that the need for experienced, credentialed coders is growing tremendously. To deal with this increased need, organizations are exploring alternatives to traditional staffing patterns. Many facilities have made the leap to at least partially electronic records, with many scanning paper records into electronic archiving systems. By making the record accessible via computer, coders do not have to be physically present in the facility to view the patient's health record. The ability to support remote coding has opened up many possibilities for staffing, including letting current employees code from home, and to use outsourcing companies.

Allowing current employees to code from home has helped organizations recruit and retain well-qualified coders. Prior to beginning a code from home program, it is recommended that specific policies and procedures are established, including maintenance of current productivity and quality standards. Other topics such as confidentiality and privacy, ownership of computers and reference materials, as well as any technology issues should be well defined. Coding remotely is not a good fit for all coding professionals and may not work well in every healthcare setting. Careful planning is essential to ensure success, but the benefits are typically worth all the planning.

Many coding companies have developed remote and electronic coding options. HIM and coding managers have opportunities to use these companies for short-term or permanent solutions. It is important to develop clear lines of communication and expectations prior to implementation of any outsourcing solution. As outside coders become familiar with the organization's internal policies and documentation issues, frequent communication will help prevent costly errors and ensure that all parties develop an ongoing, well-defined partnership.

How Changes in the System Impact Coding

One of the largest challenges faced by the coder is the nature of the ever-changing system. Each year, hundreds of diagnosis and procedure codes are added, revised, and deleted. Medicare publishes new rules governing their reimbursement system, sometimes on a quarterly basis. Insurance companies change their reimbursement policies and publish new guidelines concerning coverage for medical necessity. As the healthcare industry moves from ICD-9-CM to ICD-10-CM and ICD-10-PCS, it will be important to continue to compare data and statistics utilizing these systems. Transitioning from coding paper records to an electronic record system will create issues that may require changes in workflow and coding policies and procedures.

Coding Technology

Technology is changing many aspects of the health information profession. One of the primary areas where it has assisted in job efficiency is coding. As early as the 1980s, information technology was applied to make the coding process more effective and efficient. The type of tool used to aid in the coding process is commonly referred to as an encoder. The development of other technologies, including natural language processing (NLP), will likely have an even greater impact on the coding process.

Encoders

Encoders for ICD were developed in the early 1980s. Over the subsequent years, greater sophistication has been built into these technology solutions. An encoder is computer software that helps the coder to assign codes.

The information science and technology behind the encoding software varies from vendor to vendor. Some encoders are built using logic system techniques such as rule-based systems. Other encoding software utilizes a knowledge base approach, which incorporates automating a look-up function that provides prompts and guidance for the coding professional.

Encoders have several types of interfaces, depending on the vendor. An interface can be defined as the total component of screens, navigation, and input mechanisms used to help the end user operate the encoding software. Some encoder systems have an interface that prompts the coding professional through a series of questions. As the coder answers the questions, the encoder leads the coder to codes for diagnoses and procedures.

Alternatively, other encoders allow coders to input classification codes directly into the system and then go through a series of edit checks to ensure that only allowable code numbers are entered. In more sophisticated software systems, the encoder also prompts the coding professional to review the sequencing of the codes that have been selected in order to optimize reimbursement.

Good encoding software should include edit checks to ensure data quality. For example, an inappropriate combination of codes or inconsistent data should be flagged for the coder's attention. Encoding software is frequently linked to other information systems applications. This includes direct links to diagnosis-related group (DRG) grouper software and billing systems.

Computer-Assisted Coding

The use of encoders has become a predominant tool in the HIM department, particularly in acute care facilities. Currently, there is an even greater movement toward more complete computerization of the coding function using a supporting technology called computer-assisted coding (CAC). One prevalent definition of CAC is the use of computer software that reads clinical documentation and automatically generates a set of medical codes for review, editing, and validation by a certified coder.

There are several different types of CAC, including using software to help the physician select the correct code with processes such as drop-down boxes or the use of touch screen terminals. This is called structured input or codified input and uses menus containing clinical terms that become part of the health record documentation. This documentation then includes the information needed to assign the code.

One form of CAC is NLP. In an NLP system, digital text from online documents stored in the organization's information system is read directly by the software and then automatically coded. For example, the digital text in an online emergency department record would be interpreted automatically by the NLP system and, through the use of expert or artificial intelligence software, would automatically suggest appropriate code numbers.

This type of system will dramatically change the role of the coding professional from frontline interpreter and translator of textual data to editor, validator, or auditor of code assignments made automatically and electronically. NLP CAC is in use predominantly in the outpatient setting, where repetitive tasks can be easily automated to free the coder to focus on more complex chart review and coding assignment but is gaining usage in the inpatient setting as technology improves.

References

AHIMA. 2013. Guidelines for achieving a compliant query practice. *Journal of AHIMA*. 84(2):50–53.

AHIMA Clinical Terminology and Classification Practice Council. Key Issues Shaping Clinical Terminology and Classification. *Journal of AHIMA*. 77(7):extended online edition. http://library.ahima.org /xpedio/idcplg?IdcService=GET_HIGHLIGHT_INFO&QueryText =%28Key+issues+shaping+clinical+terminology+and+classification%29 %3Cand%3E%28xPublishSite%3Csubstring%3E%60BoK%60%29 &SortField=xPubDate&SortOrder=Desc&dDocName=bok1_031887 &HighlightType=HtmlHighlight&dWebExtension=hcsp.

American Health Information Management Association. 2013. Certification. http://www.ahima.org/certification.

American Medical Association. 2013. *CPT 2013*. Chicago. http://www .ama-assn.org/ama/pub/physician-resources/solutions-managing -your-practice/coding-billing-insurance/cpt.page.

American Hospital Association. 2013. *Coding Clinic for ICD-9-CM*. http://www.ahacentraloffice.org/.

Centers for Medicare and Medicaid Services. 2013. *ICD-10-PCS Official Guidelines for Coding and Reporting*. http://www.cms.gov/Medicare /Coding/ICD10/Downloads/pcs_2013_guidelines.pdf.

Centers for Medicare and Medicaid Services. 2013. Medicare Billing: 837I and Form CMS-1450. http://www.cms.gov/Outreach-and-Education /Medicare-Learning-Network-MLN/MLNProducts/downloads/ub04 _fact_sheet.pdf.

Centers for Medicare and Medicaid Services. 2013. Quality Improvement Organizations. http://www.cms.gov/Medicare/Quality-Initiatives -Patient-Assessment-Instruments/QualityImprovementOrgs /Current.html.

Centers for Medicare and Medicaid Services. 2013. Recovery Audit Program. http://www.cms.gov/Research-Statistics-Data-and-Systems/Monitoring -Programs/recovery-audit-program/index.html?redirect=/RAC/.

Hull, Susan. 2003. Long-term care hospital PPS creates opportunity for coding professionals. *Journal of American Health Information Management Association*. 74(6):58–60.

National Center for Health Statistics. 2013. *International Classification of Diseases, Ninth Revision, Clinical Modification.* http://www.cdc.gov /nchs/icd/icd9cm.htm.

National Center for Health Statistics. 2013. *International Classification of Diseases, Tenth Revision, Clinical Modification.* http://www.cdc.gov /nchs/icd/icd10cm.htm.

Prophet, Sue. 2008. AHIMA practice brief managing an effective query process. *Journal of AHIMA.* 79(10): 83–88.

US Department of Veterans Affairs. 2013. US Department of Veterans Affairs Health Administration Center. http://www.va.gov/hac/forbeneficiaries /champva/champva.asp.

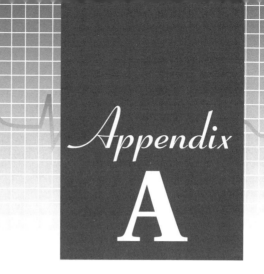

Appendix

A

AHIMA Standards of Ethical Coding

Introduction

The Standards of Ethical Coding are based on the American Health Information Management Association's (AHIMA) Code of Ethics. Both sets of principles reflect expectations of professional conduct for coding professionals involved in diagnostic or procedural coding or other health record data abstraction.

A code of ethics sets forth professional values and ethical principles and offers ethical guidelines to which professionals aspire and by which their actions can be judged. Health information management (HIM) professionals are expected to demonstrate professional values by their actions to patients, employers, members of the healthcare team, the public, and the many stakeholders they serve. A code of ethics is important in helping to guide the decision-making process and can be referenced by individuals, agencies, organizations, and bodies (such as licensing and regulatory boards, insurance providers, courts of law, government agencies, and other professional groups).

The AHIMA code of ethics (available on the AHIMA website) is relevant to all AHIMA members and credentialed HIM professionals and students, regardless of their professional functions, the settings in which they work, or the populations they serve. Coding is one of the core HIM functions, and due to the complex regulatory requirements affecting the health information coding process, coding professionals are frequently faced with ethical challenges. The AHIMA standards of ethical coding are intended to assist coding professionals and managers in decision-making processes and actions, outline expectations for making ethical decisions in the workplace, and demonstrate coding professionals' commitment to integrity during the coding process, regardless of the purpose for which the codes are being reported. They are relevant to all coding professionals and those who manage the coding function, regardless of the healthcare setting in which they work or whether they are AHIMA members or nonmembers.

These standards of ethical coding have been revised in order to reflect the current healthcare environment and modern coding practices. The previous revision was published in 1999.

Standards of Ethical Coding

Coding professionals should:

- Apply accurate, complete, and consistent coding practices for the production of high-quality healthcare data.
- Report all healthcare data elements (for example, diagnosis and procedure codes, present on admission indicator, discharge status) required for external reporting purposes (for example, reimbursement and other administrative uses, population health, quality and patient safety measurement, and research) completely and accurately, in accordance with regulatory and documentation standards and requirements and applicable official coding conventions, rules, and guidelines.
- Assign and report only the codes and data that are clearly and consistently supported by health record documentation in accordance with applicable code set and abstraction conventions, rules, and guidelines.
- Query provider (physician or other qualified healthcare practitioner) for clarification and additional documentation prior to code assignment when there is conflicting, incomplete, or ambiguous information in the health record regarding a significant reportable condition or procedure or other reportable data element dependent on health record documentation (for example, present on admission indicator).
- Refuse to change reported codes or the narratives of codes so that meanings are misrepresented.
- Refuse to participate in or support coding or documentation practices intended to inappropriately increase payment, qualify for insurance policy coverage, or skew data by means that do not comply with federal and state statutes, regulations, and official rules and guidelines.

- Facilitate interdisciplinary collaboration in situations supporting proper coding practices.
- Advance coding knowledge and practice through continuing education.
- Refuse to participate in or conceal unethical coding or abstraction practices or procedures.
- Protect the confidentiality of the health record at all times and refuse to access protected health information not required for coding-related activities (examples of coding-related activities include completion of code assignment, other health record data abstraction, coding audits, and educational purposes).
- Demonstrate behavior that reflects integrity, shows a commitment to ethical and legal coding practices, and fosters trust in professional activities.

How to Interpret the Standards of Ethical Coding

The following ethical principles are based on the core values of AHIMA, the AHIMA code of ethics, and apply to all coding professionals. Guidelines for each ethical principle include examples of behaviors and situations that can help to clarify the principle. They are not meant as a comprehensive list of all situations that can occur.

1. *Apply accurate, complete, and consistent coding practices for the production of high-quality healthcare data.*

    Coding professionals and those who manage coded data **shall**

    1.1. Support selection of appropriate diagnostic, procedure, and other types of health service related codes (for example, present on admission indicator, discharge status).

    Example:

    Policies and procedures are developed and used as a framework for the work process, and education and training is provided on their use.

    1.2. Develop and comply with comprehensive internal coding policies and procedures that are consistent with official coding rules and guidelines, reimbursement regulations, and policies and prohibit coding practices that misrepresent the patient's medical conditions and treatment provided or are not supported by the health record documentation.

Example:

Code assignment resulting in misrepresentation of facts carries significant consequences.

1.3. Participate in the development of institutional coding policies and ensure that coding policies complement, and do not conflict with, official coding rules and guidelines.

1.4. Foster an environment that supports honest and ethical coding practices resulting in accurate and reliable data.

Coding professionals **shall not**

1.5. Participate in improper preparation, alteration, or suppression of coded information.

2. *Report all healthcare data elements (for example, diagnosis and procedure codes, present on admission indicator, discharge status) required for external reporting purposes (for example,, reimbursement and other administrative uses, population health, public data reporting, quality and patient safety measurement, research) completely and accurately, in accordance with regulatory and documentation standards and requirements and applicable official coding conventions, rules, and guidelines.*

Coding professionals **shall**

2.1. Adhere to the ICD coding conventions, official coding guidelines approved by the Cooperating Parties, the CPT rules established by the American Medical Association, and any other official coding rules and guidelines established for use with mandated standard code sets.

Example:

Appropriate resource tools that assist coding professionals with proper sequencing and reporting to stay in compliance with existing reporting requirements are available and used.

2.2. Select and sequence diagnosis and procedure codes in accordance with the definitions of required data sets for applicable healthcare settings.

2.3. Comply with AHIMA's standards governing data reporting practices, including health record documentation and clinician query standards.

3. *Assign and report only the codes that are clearly and consistently supported by health record documentation in accordance with applicable code set conventions, rules, and guidelines.*

Coding professionals **shall**

3.1. Apply skills, knowledge of currently mandated coding and classification systems, and official resources to select the appropriate diagnostic and procedural codes (including applicable modifiers), and other codes representing healthcare services (including substances, equipment, supplies, or other items used in the provision of healthcare services).

Example:

Failure to research or confirm the appropriate code for a clinical condition not indexed in the classification, or reporting a code for the sake of convenience or to affect reporting for a desired effect on the results, is considered unethical.

4. *Query provider (physician or other qualified healthcare practitioner) for clarification and additional documentation prior to code assignment when there is conflicting, incomplete, or ambiguous information in the health record regarding a significant reportable condition or procedure or other reportable data element dependent on health record documentation (for example, present on admission indicator).*

Coding professionals **shall**

4.1. Participate in the development of query policies that support documentation improvement and meet regulatory, legal, and ethical standards for coding and reporting.

4.2. Query the provider for clarification when documentation in the health record that impacts an externally reportable data element is illegible, incomplete, unclear, inconsistent, or imprecise.

4.3. Use queries as a communication tool to improve the accuracy of code assignment and the quality of health record documentation, not to inappropriately increase reimbursement or misrepresent quality of care.

Example:

Policies regarding the circumstances when clinicians should be queried are designed to promote complete and accurate coding and complete documentation, regardless of whether reimbursement will be affected.

Coding professionals **shall not**

4.4. Query the provider when there is no clinical information in the health record prompting the need for a query.

Example:

Query the provider regarding the presence of gram-negative pneumonia on every pneumonia case, regardless of whether there are any clinical indications of gram-negative pneumonia documented in the record.

5. *Refuse to change reported codes or the narratives of codes so that meanings are misrepresented.*

Coding professionals **shall not**

5.1. Change the description for a diagnosis or procedure code or other reported data element so that it does not accurately reflect the official definition of that code.

Example:

The description of a code is altered in the encoding software, resulting in incorrect reporting of this code.

6. *Refuse to participate in or support coding or documentation practices intended to inappropriately increase payment, qualify for insurance policy coverage, or skew data by means that do not comply with federal and state statutes, regulations, and official rules and guidelines.*

Coding professionals **shall**

6.1. Select and sequence the codes such that the organization receives the optimal payment to which the facility is legally entitled, remembering that it is unethical and illegal to increase payment by means that contradict regulatory guidelines.

Coding professionals **shall not**

6.2. Misrepresent the patient's clinical picture through intentional incorrect coding or omission of diagnosis or procedure codes, or the addition of diagnosis or procedure codes unsupported by health record documentation, to inappropriately increase reimbursement, justify medical necessity, improve publicly reported data, or qualify for insurance policy coverage benefits.

Examples:

A patient has a health plan that excludes reimbursement for reproductive management or contraception; so rather than report the correct code for admission for tubal ligation, it is reported as a medically necessary condition with performance of a salpingectomy. The narrative descriptions of both the diagnosis and procedures reflect an admission for tubal ligation and the procedure (tubal ligation) is displayed on the record.

A code is changed at the patient's request so that the service will be covered by the patient's insurance.

6.3. Inappropriately exclude diagnosis or procedure codes in order to misrepresent the quality of care provided.

Examples:

Following a surgical procedure, a patient acquired an infection due to a break in sterile procedure; the appropriate code for the surgical complication is omitted from the claims submission to avoid any adverse outcome to the institution.

Quality outcomes are reported inaccurately in order to improve a healthcare organization's quality profile or pay-for-performance results.

7. *Facilitate interdisciplinary collaboration in situations supporting proper coding practices.*

Coding professionals **shall**

7.1. Assist and educate physicians and other clinicians by advocating proper documentation practices, further specificity, and re-sequence or include diagnoses or procedures when needed to more accurately reflect the acuity, severity, and the occurrence of events.

Example:

Failure to advocate for ethical practices that seek to represent the truth in events as expressed by the associated code sets when needed is considered an intentional disregard of these standards.

8. *Advance coding knowledge and practice through continuing education.*

Coding professionals **shall**

8.1. Maintain and continually enhance coding competency (for example, through participation in educational programs, reading official coding publications such as the Coding Clinic for ICD-9-CM, and maintaining professional certifications) in order to stay abreast of changes in codes, coding guidelines, and regulatory and other requirements.

9. *Refuse to participate in or conceal unethical coding practices or procedures.*

Coding professionals **shall**

9.1. Act in a professional and ethical manner at all times.

9.2. Take adequate measures to discourage, prevent, expose, and correct the unethical conduct of colleagues.

9.3. Be knowledgeable about established policies and procedures for handling concerns about colleagues' unethical behavior. These include policies and procedures created by AHIMA, licensing and regulatory bodies, employers, supervisors, agencies, and other professional organizations.

9.4. Seek resolution if there is a belief that a colleague has acted unethically or if there is a belief of incompetence or impairment by discussing their concerns with the colleague when feasible and when such discussion is likely to be productive. Take action through appropriate formal channels, such as contacting an accreditation or regulatory body or the AHIMA Professional Ethics Committee.

9.5. Consult with a colleague when feasible and assist the colleague in taking remedial action when there is direct knowledge of a health information management colleague's incompetence or impairment.

Coding professionals **shall not**

9.6. Participate in, condone, or be associated with dishonesty, fraud and abuse, or deception. A nonexhaustive list of examples includes

- Allowing inappropriate patterns of retrospective documentation to avoid suspension or increase reimbursement
- Assigning codes without supporting provider (physician or other qualified healthcare practitioner) documentation
- Coding when documentation does not justify the diagnoses or procedures that have been billed
- Coding an inappropriate level of service
- Miscoding to avoid conflict with others
- Adding, deleting, and altering health record documentation
- Copying and pasting another clinician's documentation without identification of the original author and date
- Knowingly reporting incorrect present on admission indicator
- Knowingly reporting incorrect patient discharge status code
- Engaging in negligent coding practices

10. *Protect the confidentiality of the health record at all times and refuse to access protected health information not required for coding-related activities (examples of coding-related activities include*

completion of code assignment, other health record data abstraction, coding audits, and educational purposes).

Coding professionals **shall**

10.1. Protect all confidential information obtained in the course of professional service, including personal, health, financial, genetic, and outcome information.

10.2. Access only that information necessary to perform their duties.

11. *Demonstrate behavior that reflects integrity, shows a commitment to ethical and legal coding practices, and fosters trust in professional activities.*

Coding professionals **shall**

11.1. Act in an honest manner and bring honor to self, peers, and the profession.

11.2. Truthfully and accurately represent their credentials, professional education, and experience.

11.3. Demonstrate ethical principles and professional values in their actions to patients, employers, other members of the healthcare team, consumers, and other stakeholders served by the healthcare data they collect and report.

Source: AHIMA House of Delegates. 2008. AHIMA Standards of Ethical Coding. http://library.ahima.org/xpedio/idcplg?IdcService=GET_HIGHLIGHT_INFO&QueryText=%28AHIMA+Standards+of+Ethical+Coding%29%3Cand%3E%28xPublishSite%3Csubstring%3E%60BoK%60%29&SortField=xPubDate&SortOrder=Desc&dDocName=bok2_001166&HighlightType=HtmlHighlight&dWebExtension=hcsp.

Appendix

B

Managing an Effective Query Process

In today's changing healthcare environment, health information management (HIM) professionals face increased demands to produce accurate coded data. Therefore, establishing and managing an effective query process is an integral component of ensuring data integrity. A query is defined as a question posed to a provider to obtain additional, clarifying documentation to improve the specificity and completeness of the data used to assign diagnosis and procedure codes in the patient's health record. Documentation can be greatly improved by a properly functioning query process.

This practice brief offers HIM professionals important components to consider in the management of an effective query process. It is intended to offer guiding principles to implement the query process while in no way prescribing what must be done.

Background

The "ICD-9-CM Official Guidelines for Coding and Reporting" are the official rules for coding and reporting ICD-9-CM. They are approved by the four organizations that make up the ICD-9-CM Cooperating Parties: the American Hospital Association, the American Health Information Management Association (AHIMA), the Centers for Medicare and Medicaid Services (CMS), and the National Center for Health Statistics. The guidelines may be used as a companion document to the official current version of the ICD-9-CM coding conventions and instructions.

The guidelines state:

A joint effort between the healthcare provider and the coding professional is essential to achieve complete and accurate documentation, code assignment, and reporting of diagnoses and procedures. These guidelines have been developed to assist both the healthcare provider and the coding professional in identifying those diagnoses and procedures that are to be reported. The importance of consistent, complete documentation in the medical record cannot be overemphasized. Without such documentation, accurate coding cannot be achieved. The entire record should be reviewed to determine the specific reason for the encounter and the conditions treated.[1]

A provider is defined as any physician or other qualified healthcare practitioner who is legally accountable for establishing the patient's diagnosis. The guidelines apply to all healthcare providers, organizations, facilities, and entities (referred to throughout this document collectively as "healthcare entities"), regardless of size and function. They are clear in their directive regarding the relationship between documentation and the accurate, consistent coding and reporting of healthcare services.

Individuals who perform the query function should be familiar with the AHIMA standards of ethical coding, which direct coders to "assign and report only the codes and data that are clearly and consistently supported by health record documentation in accordance with applicable code set and abstraction conventions, rules, and guidelines."[2] The standards further state:

Query the provider (physician or other qualified healthcare practitioner) for clarification and additional documentation prior to code assignment when there is conflicting, incomplete, or ambiguous information in the health record regarding a significant reportable condition or procedure or other reportable data element dependent on health record documentation (for example, present on admission indicator).

Organizations should establish a process for "ensuring that the physician documents in the health record any clarification or additional information resulting from communication with coding staff," according to Sue Bowman, AHIMA director of coding policy and compliance, in the book *Health Information Management Compliance: A Model Program for Healthcare Organizations.* "Communication tools between coding personnel and physicians, such as coding summary sheets, attestation forms, or coding clarification forms (for example, physician query forms), should never be used as a substitute for appropriate physician documentation in the health record."[3]

The electronic health record creates new challenges for compliance in clinical documentation. The issues to address include the use of electronic templates, generating and responding to electronic queries, and input from the appropriate staff regarding the electronic record documentation process.

The Expectations for Documentation

The primary purpose of health record documentation is continuity of patient care, serving as a means of communication among all healthcare providers. Documentation is also used to evaluate the adequacy and appropriateness of quality care, provide clinical data for research and education, and support reimbursement, medical necessity, quality of care measures, and public reporting for services rendered by a healthcare entity.[4]

Documentation and Coding

As a result of the disparity in documentation practices by providers, querying has become a common communication and educational method to advocate proper documentation practices. Queries may be made in situations such as the following:

- Clinical indicators of a diagnosis but no documentation of the condition
- Clinical evidence for a higher degree of specificity or severity
- A cause-and-effect relationship between two conditions or organism
- An underlying cause when admitted with symptoms
- Only the treatment is documented (without a diagnosis documented)
- Present on admission (POA) indicator status

Lack of accurate and complete documentation can result in the use of nonspecific and general codes, which can impact data integrity and reimbursement and present potential compliance risks.

Expectation of the Provider

According to the CMS and the Joint Commission, providers are expected to provide legible, complete, clear, consistent, precise, and reliable documentation of the patient's health history, present illness, and course of treatment. This includes observations, evidence of medical decision making in determining a diagnosis, and treatment plan, as well as the outcomes of all tests, procedures, and treatments. This documentation should be as complete and specific as possible, including information such as the level of severity, specificity of anatomical sites involved, and etiologies of symptoms.

Providers are expected to follow medical staff bylaws and assist in developing documentation and query policies and procedures. The query policy may include a statement regarding timely response and consequences for noncompliance or lack of response to queries.

Expectation of Individuals Performing the Query Function

Individuals performing the query function should follow their healthcare entity's internal policies related to documentation, querying, coding, and compliance, keeping in mind that data accuracy and integrity are fundamental HIM values. Only diagnosis codes that are clearly and consistently supported by provider documentation should be assigned and reported. A query should be initiated when there is conflicting, incomplete, or ambiguous documentation in the health record or additional information is needed for correct assignment of the POA indicator.

Expectation of the Healthcare Entity

The query process improves the quality of documentation and coding for complete clinical data capture. Queries may be initiated for all payer types regardless of the impact on reimbursement or quality reporting. The healthcare entity's documentation or compliance policies can address situations such as unnecessary queries, leading queries, repetitive overuse of queries without measureable improvement in documentation and methods for provider education.

A provider's response to a query can be documented in the progress note, discharge summary, or on the query form as a part of the formal health record. Addendums to the discharge summary or the progress note should include appropriate date and authentication.

Permanence and retention of the completed query form should be addressed in the healthcare entity's policy, taking into account applicable state and quality improvement organization guidelines. The policy should specify whether the completed query will be a permanent part of the patient's health record. If it will not be considered a permanent part of the patient's health record (for example, it might be considered a separate business record for the purpose of auditing, monitoring, and compliance), it is not subject to health record retention guidelines.

It is recommended that healthcare entities employ, educate, and train qualified individuals to perform the query process who have strong competencies in the following areas:

- Knowledge of healthcare regulations, including reimbursement and documentation requirements
- Clinical knowledge with training in pathophysiology

- Ability to read and analyze all information in a patient's health record
- Established channels of communication with providers and other clinicians
- Demonstrated skills in clinical terminology, coding, and classification systems
- Ability to apply coding conventions, official guidelines, and *Coding Clinic* advice to health record documentation

The Query Process

Who to Query

A healthcare entity's query policy should address the question of who to query. The query is directed to the provider who originated the progress note or other report in question. This could include the attending physician, consulting physician, or the surgeon. In most cases, a query for abnormal test results would be directed to the attending physician.

Documentation from providers involved in the care and treatment of the patient is appropriate for code assignment; however, a query may be necessary if the documentation conflicts with that of another provider. If such a conflict exists, the attending physician is queried for clarification, as that provider is ultimately responsible for the final diagnosis.

When to Query

Providers should be queried whenever there is conflicting, ambiguous, or incomplete information in the health record regarding any *significant* reportable condition or procedure.

Queries are not necessary for every discrepancy or unaddressed issue in physician documentation. Healthcare entities should develop policies and procedures that clarify which clinical conditions and documentation situations warrant a request for physician clarification. Insignificant or irrelevant findings may not warrant a query regarding the assignment of an additional diagnosis code, for example. Entities must balance the value of collecting marginal data against the administrative burden of obtaining the additional documentation.

Healthcare entities could consider a policy in which queries may be appropriate when documentation in the patient's record fails to meet one of the following five criteria:

1. *Legibility*: This might include an illegible handwritten entry in the provider's progress notes, and the reader cannot determine the provider's assessment on the date of discharge.

2. *Completeness*: This might include a report indicating abnormal test results without notation of the clinical significance of these results (for example, an x-ray shows a compression fracture of lumbar vertebrae in a patient with osteoporosis and no evidence of injury).

3. *Clarity*: This might include patient diagnosis noted without statement of a cause or suspected cause (for example, the patient is admitted with abdominal pain, fever, and chest pain and no underlying cause or suspected cause is documented).

4. *Consistency*: This might include a disagreement between two or more treating providers with respect to a diagnosis (for example, the patient presents with shortness of breath; the pulmonologist documents pneumonia as the cause, and the attending documents congestive heart failure as the cause).

5. *Precision*: This might include an instance where clinical reports and clinical condition suggest a more specific diagnosis than is documented (for example, congestive heart failure is documented when an echocardiogram and the patient's documented clinical condition on admission suggest acute or chronic diastolic congestive heart failure).

Healthcare entities may design their query programs to be concurrent, retrospective, postbill, or a combination of any of these. Concurrent queries are initiated while the patient is still present. Retrospective queries are initiated after discharge and before the bill is submitted; postbill queries are initiated after the bill has been submitted.

Concurrent queries are initiated "real time," during the course of the patient encounter or hospitalization, at the time the documentation is naturally done. They thus encourage more timely, accurate, and reliable responses. Retrospective queries are effective in cases where additional information is available in the health record, in short stays where concurrent review was not completed, or whenever a concurrent query process is not feasible.

Postbill queries are initiated after the claim is submitted or remittance advice is paid. Postbill queries generally occur as a result of an audit or other internal monitor. Healthcare entities can develop a policy regarding whether they will generate postbill queries and the time frame following claims generation that queries may be initiated. They may consider the following three concepts in the development of a postbill (including query) policy:

- Applying normal course of business guidelines[5]
- Using payer-specific rules on rebilling time frames
- Determining reliability of query response over time

When Not to Query

Codes assigned to clinical data should be clearly and consistently supported by provider documentation. Providers often make clinical diagnoses that may not appear to be consistent with test results. For example, the provider may make a clinical determination that the patient has pneumonia when the results of the chest x-ray may be negative. Queries should not be used to question a provider's clinical judgment, but rather to clarify documentation when it fails to meet any of the five criteria listed earlier—legibility, completeness, clarity, consistency, or precision.

A query may not be appropriate simply because the clinical information or clinical picture does not appear to support the documentation of a condition or procedure (for example, documentation of acute respiratory failure in a patient whose laboratory findings do not appear to support this diagnosis). In situations where the provider's documented diagnosis does not appear to be supported by clinical findings, a healthcare entity's policies can provide guidance on a process for addressing the issue without querying the attending physician.

The Query Format

It is recommended that the healthcare entity's policy address the query format. A query generally includes the following information:

- Patient name
- Admission date and/or date of service
- Health record number
- Account number
- Date query initiated
- Name and contact information of the individual initiating the query
- Statement of the issue in the form of a question along with clinical indicators specified from the chart (for example, history and physical states urosepsis, lab reports WBC of 14,400. Emergency department report fever of 102)

It is not advisable to record queries on handwritten sticky notes, scratch paper, or other notes that can be removed and discarded. The preferred formats for capturing the query include facility-approved query form, facsimile transmission, electronic communication on secure e-mail, or secure IT messaging system.

Verbal queries have become more common as a component of the concurrent query process. The desired result of a verbal query is documentation by the provider that supports the coding of a condition, diagnosis, or procedure. Therefore, entities should develop specific policies to clearly address this practice and avoid potential compliance risks.

It is recommended that queries be written with precise language, identifying clinical indications from the health record, and asking the provider to make a clinical interpretation of these facts based on his or her professional judgment of the case. Queries that appear to lead the provider to document a particular response could result in allegations of inappropriate upcoding. The query format should not sound presumptive, directing, prodding, probing, or as though the provider is being led to make an assumption.

Examples of leading queries include:

Dr. Smith—Based on your documentation, this patient has anemia and was transfused two units of blood. Also, there was a 10-point drop in hematocrit following surgery. Please document "Acute Blood Loss Anemia," as this patient clearly meets the clinical criteria for this diagnosis.

Dr. Jones—This patient has COPD and is on oxygen every night at home and has been on continuous oxygen since admission. Please document "Chronic Respiratory Failure."

In these examples, the provider is not given any documentation option other than the specific diagnosis requested. The statements are directive, indicating what the provider should document, rather than querying the provider for his or her professional determination of the clinical facts. In the first example, the statement "the patient has anemia" may be presumptive, and the statement "please document 'acute blood loss anemia'" is directive and clearly leading the provider. In the second example, the provider is inappropriately asked to document chronic respiratory failure.

Examples of the above queries correctly written could include the following:

Dr. Smith—In your progress note on 6/20, you documented anemia and ordered transfusion of two units of blood. Also, according to the lab work done on xx/xx, the patient had a 10-point drop in hematocrit following surgery. Based on these indications, please document, in the discharge summary, the type of anemia you were treating.

Dr. Jones—This patient has COPD and is on oxygen every night at home and has been on continuous oxygen since admission. Based on these indications, please indicate if you were treating one of the following diagnoses:

- Chronic Respiratory Failure
- Acute Respiratory Failure
- Acute on Chronic Respiratory Failure
- Hypoxia
- Unable to determine
- Other:_____

The introduction of new information not previously documented in the medical record is inappropriate in a provider query. For example,
Dr. Harvey—According to the patient's emergency room record from last week, the patient was placed on antibiotics for cellulitis of her leg. If the patient is still taking antibiotics, please document the cellulitis.

In this case, if this diagnosis was not documented in the current admission and is not affecting the patient's care, it does not meet the definition of a secondary diagnosis.[6] Querying for this new information, which does not meet coding and reporting requirements, is inappropriate.

In general, query forms should not be designed to ask questions about a diagnosis or procedure that can be responded to in a yes/no fashion. The exception is POA queries when the diagnosis has already been documented.

It is recommended that healthcare entities address the issue of yes/no queries in their policies. When setting this policy, the entity should consider the compliance risk. In general, it is a much safer practice to ask the provider to document the diagnosis he or she is agreeing to. Concerns about yes/no queries are less of an issue if the entity requires the provider to document the diagnosis in the health record rather than relying on the query form for the final documentation.

Multiple choice formats that employ checkboxes may be used as long as all clinically reasonable choices are listed, regardless of the impact on reimbursement or quality reporting. The choices should also include an "other" option, with a line that allows the provider to add free text. Providers should also be given the choice of "unable to determine." This format is designed to make multiple choice questions as open ended as possible.

A single query form can be used to address multiple questions. If it is, a distinct question should be asked for each issue (for example, if three questions exist based on clinical indications in the health record, there should be three distinct questions clearly identified on the query form).

For example, insulin-dependent diabetes with high blood sugars on admission is documented in a patient with renal failure. The three questions identified on the query might be related to type of diabetes (type I or II or secondary), relationship of diabetes to renal failure, and whether the diabetes is controlled or uncontrolled.

Finally, the query should never indicate that a particular response would favorably or unfavorably affect reimbursement or quality reporting.

Methods of Auditing and Monitoring

Healthcare entities should consider establishing an auditing and monitoring program as a means to improve their query processes. They can consider several methods for this ongoing process.

Queries can be reviewed retrospectively to ensure that they are completed according to documented policies. This might include reviewing

- That the query was necessary
- That the language used in the query was not leading or otherwise inappropriate
- That the query did not introduce new information from the health record

Based on the results of this review, the healthcare entity may need to identify follow-up actions. For example, cases identified as inappropriate queries resulting in inaccurate code assignment will require that codes be corrected at the level supported by the documentation without the leading query. Inappropriate queries should be tracked and trended, followed by appropriate education and training.

In order for the query process to be effective, auditing and monitoring should be conducted on a regular basis. This process can include a representative sample of total queries as well as a sampling by individuals initiating the query. Effective elements of an auditing and monitoring program include the following:

- Auditing for percentage of negative and positive provider responses. A high negative response rate may indicate overuse of the query by the coding staff; a high positive response rate may indicate a pattern of incomplete documentation that needs further investigation.
- Auditing the format of query forms. Discovery of inappropriate query formats can be used as an educational tool for coding staff.
- Auditing of individual providers to indicate improvement in health record documentation. Improvement in documentation should result in a decreased number of queries for an individual provider.
- Auditing of high-risk or problem diagnoses. The results may determine whether additional education resulted in a decreased number of queries for a particular diagnosis.

Auditing and monitoring programs should establish the data fields to be collected and reported. When reviewing both performance measures and compliance monitors, the errors related to documentation will become apparent.

Healthcare entities should have a process in place to support and educate the staff involved in conducting provider queries. Ongoing education and training is a key component of the auditing and monitoring process.

Conclusion

HIM professionals are constantly challenged to improve the accuracy of coded data to meet regulatory, state, and federal requirements. In addition, electronic records pose new challenges in the collection and maintenance of quality data.

The quality of coding is driven directly by the documentation contained in the patient's health record. Establishing and managing a query process can be an effective tool to improve clinical documentation and thereby increase the accuracy of coded data. Typically, both concurrent and retrospective query processes are needed. An effective query process, using an appropriate format, will enable the facility to obtain needed documentation without compromising coding compliance standards.

Since the query process has become a tool to improve provider documentation, it is critical that the design of these processes be maintained with legal, regulatory, and ethical issues in mind. Healthcare entities can create and maintain a compliant query process by

- Creating comprehensive policies and procedures for query processes
- Generating queries only when documentation is conflicting, incomplete, or ambiguous
- Conducting auditing and monitoring activities to determine the effectiveness of the query process
- Providing education and training for the staff involved in conducting provider queries

Notes

1. Centers for Medicare and Medicaid Services and the National Center for Health Statistics. ICD-9-CM Official Guidelines for Coding and Reporting. www.cdc.gov/nchs/datawh/ftpserv/ftpicd9/ftpicd9.htm#guidelines.
2. AHIMA. 2008 Standards of Ethical Coding. www.ahima.org/infocenter/guidelines.
3. Prophet, Sue. 2002. *Health Information Management Compliance: A Model Program for Healthcare Organizations*. 2d edition. (Chicago, IL: AHIMA).
4. For the purposes of this practice brief, *healthcare entity* encompasses all providers: short-term acute care hospitals; long-term acute care hospitals; skilled nursing facility and hospice; inpatient and outpatient psychiatric and rehabilitation; home health; hospital-based outpatient and clinic; and all professional providers such as physician practice as

well as any other healthcare entity or professional provider that serves patient care solo or as part of a corporation. The healthcare entity uses the same policies and procedures throughout the components of the organization.

5. Normal course of business guidelines include ensuring that the postbill query process is conducted in the healthcare entity's normal time frame for completing health records in accordance with medical staff bylaws and rules and regulations for health record completion.

6. For reporting purposes, the term *other diagnoses* is interpreted as additional conditions that affect patient care in terms of requiring clinical evaluation, therapeutic treatment, diagnostic procedures, extended length of hospital stay, or increased nursing care and monitoring. Uniform Hospital Discharge Data Set item 11-b defines other diagnoses as "all conditions that coexist at the time of admission, that develop subsequently, or that affect the treatment received and/or the length of stay. Diagnoses that related to an earlier episode which have no bearing on the current hospital stay are to be excluded."

The information contained in this practice brief reflects the consensus opinion of the professionals who developed it. It has not been validated through scientific research.

This practice brief updates the 2001 practice brief "Developing a Physician Query Process," with a continued focus on compliance.

Source: AHIMA. 2008. (October) Managing an effective query process. *Journal of AHIMA* 79(10):83–88.

Index

A

AFDC program. *See* Aid to Families with Dependent Children (AFDC) program
Agency for Healthcare Research and Quality (AHRQ), 80–82
AHA. *See* American Hospital Association (AHA)
AHIMA. *See* American Health Information Management Association (AHIMA)
AHIMA Professional Ethics Committee, 98
AHRQ. *See* Agency for Healthcare Research and Quality (AHRQ)
Aid to Families with Dependent Children (AFDC) program, 54
Alphabetic Index, 17
   use of, 27–28
AMA. *See* American Medical Association (AMA)
Ambulatory payment classification (APC) system
   annual review, 52
   CCI edits, 51–52
   description, 45
   discounting computation, 51
   grouping codes in, 46
   inpatient only procedures, 51
   medical visits, 52
   packaging, 46
   status indicators, 46–50
   weights and payments, 51
American Health Information Management Association (AHIMA), 5, 64, 77, 78
   code of ethics, 91
   standards of ethical coding, 91–99, 102
American Hospital Association (AHA), 5
   coding process, 73

American Medical Association (AMA), 3, 94
   coding process, 73
Appendices in CPT codes, 27
Audit plan, 79
Auditing, compliance plan, 66

B

Balanced Budget Act of 1997, 18, 44, 76–77
Balanced Budget Refinement Act of 1999, 44
Barre-Guillain Syndrome, 8
Beneficiaries, 33
   LOS, 41
Benefits Improvement and Protection Act of 2000, 44
Billing forms, 78
   CMS-1500 form, 58, 59
   description, 57–58
   hospital billing formats, 58, 60
Billing patterns
   coding and, 68
   utilization and, 68
Blue Cross and Blue Shield program, 56–57

C

CAC. *See* Computer-assisted coding (CAC)
CAHIIM. *See* Commission on Accreditation for Health Informatics and Information Management Education (CAHIIM)
Case managers, PPS, 36
Case-mix index (CMI), 43, 67–68
Category codes, 27
CC. *See* Complication or comorbidity (CC)
CCA examination. *See* Certified Coding Associate (CCA) examination

CCI edits. *See* Correct coding initiative (CCI) edits

CCS examination. *See* Certified Coding Specialists (CCS) examination

CCS-P examination. *See* Certified Coding Specialist-Physician Based (CCS-P) examination

CDIP. *See* Clinical Documentation Improvement Program (CDIP)

CDSs. *See* Clinical documentation specialists (CDSs)

Centers for Medicare and Medicaid Services (CMS), 5, 61, 64, 103
  Medicaid Eligibility Summary, 54
  Medicare program, 33
  pay-for-performance initiatives, 81–82

Certified Coding Associate (CCA) examination, 84

Certified Coding Specialist-Physician Based (CCS-P) examination, 84–85

Certified Coding Specialists (CCS) examination, 84–85

CF. *See* Conversion factor (CF)

Civilian Health and Medical Program of the Department of Veterans Affairs (CHAMPVA), 55, 56

Clinical decision support, healthcare data, 82

Clinical Documentation Improvement Program (CDIP), 79–80

Clinical documentation specialists (CDSs), 80

Clot buster drugs, 52

CMI. *See* Case-mix index (CMI)

CMS. *See* Centers for Medicare and Medicaid Services (CMS)

CMS-1450 form, 58, 60

CMS-1500 form, 57–59

COBRA of 1986. *See* Consolidated Omnibus Budget Reconciliation Act (COBRA) of 1986

Code assignment, 94

Code of ethics, 91

Coded data, uses of, 80–82

Codified input, CAC, 87

Coding Clinic for ICD-9-CM, 97

Coding compliance
  components of compliance plan, 65–69
  fraud and abuse, 61–64
  healthcare quality improvement organizations, 69–71
  policies and procedures, 64–65
  RACs, 64
  standards of ethical coding, 64

Coding process
  description, 73
  inpatient, 74–75
  linking diagnosis to procedure, 76–77
  outpatient, 75–76
  physician query process, 77–79
  quality assessment for, 79–82
  secondary diagnosis, 77
  steps in, 73–74
  technologies, 86–87

Coding professionals, 28
  challenges, 86
  examinations for, 84–85
  RHIAs, 83–84
  RHITs, 83
  shortage of, 85–86

Coding systems
  CPT. *See* current procedural terminology (CPT)
  data sets, 2–3
  defined and explained, 1–2
  documentation and, 103
  HCPCS. *See* Healthcare Common Procedure Coding System (HCPCS)
  ICD-11, 19
  ICD-9-CM. *See International Classification of Diseases, Ninth Revision, Clinical Modification* (ICD-9-CM)
  ICD-10-CM. *See International Classification of Diseases, Tenth Revision, Clinical Modification* (ICD-10-CM)
  issues in coding diagnosis, 17–18
  medical necessity, 18

Colonoscopy, CPT/HCPCS code choices for, 21

Combination codes in ICD-10-CM, 12
Commercial group medical insurance
    plan, 56–57
Commission on Accreditation
    for Health Informatics and
    Information Management
    Education (CAHIIM), 83
Communication, 66
Compliance plan
    auditing and monitoring, 66
    communication, 66
    corrective action and follow-up,
        66–69
    designation of compliance officer, 65
    documentation requirements, 69
    guidance, 63–64
    training and education, 66
Compliance Program Guidance
    (CPG), 65
Complication or comorbidity
    (CC), 38–39
    exclusion list, 39
Comprehensive internal coding policies
    and procedures, 93
Computer-assisted coding (CAC), 87
Concurrent query process, 106, 107
Consolidated Omnibus Budget
    Reconciliation Act (COBRA) of
    1986, 57
Conventions, coding, 26
Conversion factor (CF), 53
Coordination of care, 31
Correct coding initiative (CCI) edits,
    51–52
Corrective action and follow-up, 66–67
Cost outlier, 40
Counseling, 31
CPG. See Compliance Program
    Guidance (CPG)
CPT. See Current procedural
    terminology (CPT)
CPT Advisory Committee, 24
Current procedural terminology (CPT),
    23–24
    alphabetic index, use of, 27–28
    appendices, 27
    category codes, 27

code choices for colonoscopy, 21
coding conventions, 26
E/M coding section. See Evaluation
    and Management (E/M) codes
modifiers, 28–29
overview of structure, 25–26
procedure codes, 3
purpose and use, 24–25
rules for, 27–28, 94
Cystoscopy, 24
Cystourethroscopy, 24

D
Data integrity, 101
Denials
    claims, 68
    inappropriate, 69
    spreadsheet, example of, 68
Department of Health and Human
    Services (HHS), 2, 61
Designation of Compliance Officer, 65
Diagnosis codes, assignment of, 32
Diagnosis-related group (DRG) system,
    4, 37–38, 67
    relative weight, 39–41
DME. See Durable medical equipment
    (DME)
DMERC. See Durable medical
    equipment regional carrier
    (DMERC)
Documentation guidelines, CMS, 31–32
DRG system. See Diagnosis-related
    group (DRG) system
Durable medical equipment (DME),
    20, 34
Durable medical equipment regional
    carrier (DMERC), 34

E
Effective compliance program, 63–64
Effective query process, management
    of, 101–3, 105–9
    auditing and monitoring, methods
        of, 109–10
    documentation, expectations for,
        103–5
Electronic health record (EHR), 19, 102–3

E/M codes. *See* Evaluation and
  Management (E/M) codes
Encoders, 86–87
End-stage renal disease (ESRD), 33
EOB. *See* Explanation of Benefits (EOB)
Error reports, claims denials and, 68
ESRD. *See* End-stage renal
  disease (ESRD)
Evaluation and Management (E/M)
  codes, 52
  documentation guidelines, 31–32
  extent of examination, 30
  extent of patient history, 29–30
  medical decision making, 30–31
  new versus established patient, 31
  notes, 32
Expanded Problem Focused, 30
Explanation of Benefits (EOB), 79

F
FBI. *See* Federal Bureau of
  Investigation (FBI)
FCA. *See* Federal Civil False Claims
  Act (FCA)
Federal Bureau of Investigation
  (FBI), 61
Federal Civil False Claims Act (FCA), 62
Federal poverty level (FPL), 54
Fee-for-service reimbursement plan, 35
FI. *See* Fiscal intermediary (FI)
FIM-FRGs. *See* Functional
  independence measures–
  functional-related groups
  (FIM-FRGs)
Fiscal intermediary (FI), 33–34
Follow-up, corrective action and, 66–67
FPL. *See* Federal poverty level (FPL)
Frequency of Service, 46
Functional independence measures–
  functional-related groups
  (FIM-FRGs), 45

G
General multisystem examination, 30
Geographic practice cost index
  (GPCI), 53
Group medical insurance plans, 56–57

Grouper software
  annual updates, 41–42
  case-mix index, 43
  description, 41
  HAC, 42–43
  MS-DRG, 42
  severity of illness, 42

H
HAC. *See* Hospital-acquired
  condition (HAC)
HCFA. *See* Health Care Financing
  Administration (HCFA)
HCPCS. *See* Healthcare Common
  Procedure Coding System
  (HCPCS)
Health Care Financing Administration
  (HCFA), 20
Health information management
  (HIM), 91
  professionals, 83, 101
*Health Information Management
  Compliance: A Model Program
  for Healthcare Organizations*
  (Bowman), 102
Health Insurance Portability and
  Accountability Act (HIPAA), 2, 14, 57
Health insurance prospective payment
  system (HIPPS) codes, 45
Health record
  documentation, primary purpose of, 103
  protecting confidentiality of, 98–99
Healthcare
  data elements report, 92, 94
  facilities, types of, 63
  quality improvement organizations,
    Medicare quality initiative, 69–71
Healthcare Common Procedure Coding
  System (HCPCS)
  code choices for colonoscopy, 21
  level I, 5
  level II modifiers, 23
  level II section titles, 21–22
  National Panel, 21
  overview of structure, 20–23
  procedure codes, 3
  purpose and use, 20

Healthcare entities, 102, 106, 110
  documentation/compliance
    policies, 104
  expectation of, 104
  internal policies, 104
  policy, 107
  query policy, 105
HHS. *See* Department of Health and
    Human Services (HHS)
High-quality healthcare data
    production, coding practices for,
    93–94
HIPAA. *See* Health Insurance Portability
    and Accountability Act (HIPAA)
HIPPS codes. *See* Health insurance
    prospective payment system
    (HIPPS) codes
Hospital inpatient coding, 18
Hospital reimbursement program,
    56–57
Hospital Value-based Purchasing
    Program, 69
Hospital-acquired condition (HAC),
    42–43

I
ICD-11 coding system, 19
ICD-9-CM. *See International
    Classification of Diseases, Ninth
    Revision, Clinical Modification*
    (ICD-9-CM)
ICD-10-CM. *See International
    Classification of Diseases, Tenth
    Revision, Clinical Modification*
    (ICD-10-CM)
ICD-9-CM Cooperating Parties, 101
ICD-9-CM Official Guidelines for
    Coding and Report, 101
ICD-10-PCS. *See International
    Classification of Diseases, Tenth
    Revision, Procedure Coding
    System* (ICD-10-PCS)
Inappropriate denials, 69
Inappropriate queries, 110
Inpatient coding process, 74–75
Inpatient hospitals, quality measures
    for, 70–71

Inpatient only procedures, APC
    system, 51
Inpatient Prospective Payment System
    (IPPS), 19, 40–41, 43–45
Inpatient psychiatric facility (IPF), 45
Inpatient rehabilitation facilities (IRFs),
    44–45
Inpatient rehabilitation facilities-
    patient assessment instrument
    (IRF-PAI), 45
Inpatient rehabilitation hospital PPS,
    44–45
Insurance programs
  group medical insurance plans,
    56–57
  Medicaid, 54
  military programs, 54–56
*International Classification of Diseases,
    Ninth Revision, Clinical
    Modification* (ICD-9-CM)
  classification system, 37
  diagnosis and procedure codes, 3
  to ICD-10-CM, transition from, 6
  overview of, 17
*International Classification of Diseases,
    Tenth Revision, Clinical
    Modification* (ICD-10-CM), 3–4
  categories, subcategories, and
    subclassifications, 9–10
  chapter titles in, 8–9
  coding conventions, 10–11
  coding guidelines, 5–6
  combination codes, 12
  cooperating parties, 5
  identify subterms, 8
  locating main term, 7–8
  nonessential modifier, 8
  nonspecific/residual codes, 10
  not elsewhere classified and not
    otherwise specified, 12
  overview of structure, 6–7
  purpose, 4
  revisions to, 19
  sequencing of codes, 13
  steps of coding, 12–13
  transition from ICD-9-CM to, 6
  using the tabular list, 8–9

International Classification of Diseases, Tenth Revision, Procedure Coding System (ICD-10-PCS)
characters of, 16
coding guidelines, 14
overview of structure, 15–16
purpose and use, 14
sections of, 15
IPF. *See* Inpatient psychiatric facility (IPF)
IPPS. *See* Inpatient Prospective Payment System (IPPS)
IRF-PAI. *See* Inpatient rehabilitation facilities-patient assessment instrument (IRF-PAI)
IRFs. *See* Inpatient rehabilitation facilities (IRFs)

J
J codes, 21
Joint Commission, 103

L
LCDs. *See* Local coverage determinations (LCDs)
Length of stay (LOS), 41
LMRPs. *See* Local medical review policies (LMRPs)
Local coverage determinations (LCDs), 34
Local medical review policies (LMRPs), 34
Long-term acute care hospitals (LTCHs), 44
LOS. *See* Length of stay (LOS)
LTCHs. *See* Long-term acute care hospitals (LTCHs)

M
MA. *See* Medicare Advantage (MA)
MACs. *See* Medicare Administrative Contractors (MACs)
Major complications/comorbidities (MCCs), 39
Malpractice cost (MP), 53
MA-PD. *See* Medicare Advantage-Prescription Drug (MA-PD)

MCCs. *See* Major complications/comorbidities (MCCs)
Medicaid, 54
Medicaid Management Information System, 24
Medical decision making, 30–31
evidence of, 103
Medical plans, major, 56
Medicare
description, 33–34
DRG relative weight, 39–41
enrollees, 33
grouper software, 41–43
inpatient PPSs, 43–45
MS-DRGs, 43
outpatient PPSs, 45–52
PPS, 35–38
principal diagnosis, 38
quality initiative, 69–71
reimbursement system, 86
secondary diagnoses, 38–39
Medicare Administrative Contractors (MACs), 34
Medicare Advantage (MA), 34–35
Medicare Advantage-Prescription Drug (MA-PD), 35
Medicare inpatient acute care PPS, structure and organization of, 37–38
Medicare, Medicaid, and SCHIP Benefits Improvement and Protection Act of 2000, 44–45
Medicare Modernization Act, 69
Medicare Part A, 34
Medicare Part B, 34
Medicare Part C, 34–35
Medicare Part D, 35
Medicare Prescription Drug Plan, 35
Medicare Provider Analysis and Review (MedPAR) database, 44
Medicare Severity-adjusted Diagnosis-Related Groups (MS-DRGs), 37
uses of, 43
Medicare severity-adjusted long-term care hospital prospective payment system (MS-LTCH-PPS), 44

MedPAR database. *See* Medicare Provider Analysis and Review (MedPAR) database
Military programs, insurance, 54–56
Modifiers
   in CPT, 28–29
   HCPCS level II, 23
   nonessential, 8
Monitoring
   auditing and, 66
   claims denials and error reports, 68
   coding and DRG Changes, 68
   program plan, 79
MP. *See* Malpractice cost (MP)
MS-DRGs. *See* Medicare Severity-adjusted Diagnosis-Related Groups (MS-DRGs)
MS-LTCH-PPS. *See* Medicare severity-adjusted long-term care hospital prospective payment system (MS-LTCH-PPS)

N
"Naming" system, 24
National Center for Health Statistics (NCHS), 5
National Codes, 20
National coverage determinations (NCDs), 33
National Provider Identifier (NPI), 58
National Uniform Billing Committee (NUBC), 57, 58
National Uniform Claim Committee (NUCC), 57
Natural language processing (NLP) system, 87
NCDs. *See* National coverage determinations (NCDs)
NCHS. *See* National Center for Health Statistics (NCHS)
NLP system. *See* Natural language processing (NLP) system
Nomenclature system, 24
Nonprofit group medical insurance plan, 56–57
Nonspecific codes, 10

NPI. *See* National Provider Identifier (NPI)
NUBC. *See* National Uniform Billing Committee (NUBC)
NUCC. *See* National Uniform Claim Committee (NUCC)

O
OCE. *See* Outpatient Code Editor (OCE)
Office of the Inspector General (OIG)
   guidance for compliance programs, 62
   work plan, 62–63
Omnibus Budget Reconciliation Act, 24
OPPS system. *See* Outpatient Prospective Payment System (OPPS)
Outliers, cost, 40
Outpatient Code Editor (OCE), 51
Outpatient coding process, 75–76
Outpatient Prospective Payment System (OPPS), 45–52
   billing, 29

P
Patient assessment instrument (PAI), 45
Patient safety evaluation, 81
Patient Safety Indicators (PSIs), 81
Patients
   level of care, 31
   new versus established, 31
   signs and symptoms, 17
Pay-for-performance initiatives, 81–82
Payment rates, 36
PDP. *See* Prescription drug plan (PDP)
PE. *See* Practice expense (PE)
Physical examination, 30
Physicians
   payment for, 52–53
   professional service, 29
PIP-DCG algorithm. *See* Principal inpatient diagnostic cost group (PIP-DCG) algorithm
POA. *See* Present on admission (POA)
Post-acute care transfer policy, 40–41
Postbill policy, development of, 106
Postbill queries, 106

PPS. *See* Prospective payment
  system (PPS)
Practice expense (PE), 53
Preferred payment plan, 56
Preprinted forms, 75, 76
Prescription drug plan (PDP), 35
Present on admission (POA), 42
Primary diagnosis, 75
Principal diagnosis, 38
Principal inpatient diagnostic cost
  group (PIP-DCG) algorithm, 35
Prospective payment system (PPS)
  characteristics, 36–37
  description, 35–36
  inpatient rehabilitation hospital,
    44–45
  IPF, 45
  long-term acute care, 44
  Medicare inpatient acute care, 37–38
  Medicare outpatient, 45–52
  RBRVS, 52–53
PSIs. *See* Patient Safety Indicators (PSIs)
Public health surveillance, 82
Punctuation marks, CPT codes, 25

Q
QIO. *See* Quality improvement
  organizations (QIO)
Quality
  of care assessment, 80–82
  measures for inpatient hospitals,
    70–71
Quality assessment for coding process,
  79–82
  CDIP, 79–80
  coded data uses, 80–82
  description, 79
Quality improvement organizations
  (QIO), healthcare, 69–71
Queries, 95, 103–4, 107, 110
  format, 107–9
  policy, 104
  postbill queries, 106
  retrospective queries, 106
Query function, 102
  expectation of individuals
    performing, 104

R
RA. *See* Remittance Advice (RA)
RACs. *See* Recovery audit contractors
  (RACs)
RBRVS. *See* Resource-Based Relative
  Value System/Scale (RBRVS)
Recovery audit contractors (RACs),
  17, 64
Registered Health Information
  Administrators (RHIAs), 83–84
Registered Health Information
  Technicians (RHITs), 83
Reimbursement
  billing forms, 57–60
  group medical insurance plans,
    56–57
  insurance programs, 53–56
  Medicare. *See* Medicare
  physicians payment, 52–53
Relative value units (RVUs), 53
Relative weight, DRG
  description, 39–40
  outliers, 40
  post-acute care transfer policy,
    40–41
Remittance Advice (RA), 79
Residual codes, 10
Resource-Based Relative Value System/
  Scale (RBRVS), 52–53
Retrospective queries, 106
Returned to the provider (RTP), 68
RHIAs. *See* Registered Health
  Information Administrators
  (RHIAs)
RHITs. *See* Registered Health
  Information Technicians (RHITs)
Risk-adjustment methodologies, 81
RTP. *See* Returned to the provider (RTP)
RVUs. *See* Relative value units (RVUs)

S
Scrubber, software program, 78
Secondary diagnosis coding, 38–39,
  42, 77
Sections, CPT code book, 25
Sequencing of codes, 13
Social Security Act, 33, 37, 54

Software program, scrubber, 78
SSI. *See* Supplemental Security Income
(SSI)
Standards of ethical coding, 64, 91–93
interpreting, 93–99
Status indicators, APC system, 46–50
Structured input, CAC, 87
Supplemental Security Income (SSI), 54
Symbols, CPT codes, 25

T
Tabular List, 17
Tax Equity and Fiscal Responsibility Act
(TEFRA), 37
Temporary national codes, 21–23
Training and education, compliance
plans, 66
Transfer policy, post-acute care
settings, 41
TRICARE, 55–56
TRICARE Extra, 55
TRICARE for Life, 55
TRICARE Plus, 55

TRICARE Prime, 55
TRICARE Standard, 55

U
UB-04. *See* Uniform Billing-04
(UB-04)
UHDDS. *See* Uniform Hospital
Discharge Data Set (UHDDS)
Uniform Billing-04 (UB-04), 57, 58, 60
Uniform Hospital Discharge Data Set
(UHDDS)
guidelines, 13
principal diagnosis, 38
secondary diagnosis, 38–39
Utilization review (UR) professionals, 36

V
VA. *See* Veterans Administration (VA)
Verbal queries, 107
Veterans Administration (VA), 55

W
Wage index, 40